HEALTH CARE
in Canada

ANTONIA MAIONI

D1202465

ISSUES IN CANADA

OXFORD
UNIVERSITY PRESS

OXFORD
UNIVERSITY PRESS

Oxford University Press is a department of the University of Oxford.
It furthers the University's objective of excellence in research, scholarship,
and education by publishing worldwide. Oxford is a registered trade mark of
Oxford University Press in the UK and in certain other countries.

Published in Canada by
Oxford University Press
8 Sampson Mews, Suite 204,
Don Mills, Ontario M3C 0H5 Canada

www.oupcanada.com

Library and Archives Canada Cataloguing in Publication

Maioni, Antonia, author
Health care in Canada / Antonia Maioni.
(Issues in Canada)

Includes bibliographical references and index.
ISBN 978-0-19-900338-9 (pbk.)

1. Medical care--Canada. I. Title. II. Series: Issues in Canada

RA395.C3M349 2014   362.10971   C2014-90340

Cover image: nyul/iStockphoto

Oxford University Press is committed to our environment.
This book is printed on Forest Stewardship Council® certified paper
and comes from responsible sources.

MIX
Paper from
responsible sources
FSC
www.fsc.org   FSC® C004071

Printed and bound in Canada

1 2 3 4 — 18 17 16 15

Contents

Preface

The inspiration for this book came from a well-known—but unlikely—source: Ken Dryden. Some of you may remember him as a hockey legend and championship goalie for the Montreal Canadiens, others for his management experience with the Toronto Maple Leafs in the National Hockey League, and still others as a Member of Parliament and leadership contender for the Liberal Party of Canada.

After his political career, Ken came to teach at the McGill Institute for the Study of Canada. He designed a class around the innovative idea of "thinking the future" and invited several professors to speak to the students. Not, as we are used to, about our research per se, but about the personal journey that had led us to that research and to where we are now.

So, out went the PowerPoint presentation and the canned lecture. As I prepared for my talk, what became evident was that the study of health care was, for all intents and purposes, essentially the study of Canada itself. To trace the historical evolution of health care as a public policy and as a political debate was to understand how Canada works: its political institutions, constitutional origins, political organization, ideological cleavages, and evolving values. And an understanding of health care required the unravelling of larger questions about government spending, the role of a modern state, and the crucial elements of the relationship between state and society.

The aim of this book is to provide an introduction to that understanding, by attempting to make clear the facts and figures of health care in Canada. It does not take an ideological position or try to hammer home a particular side of the health debate. Instead, it tells the story of how the public insurance systems in Canada evolved over time, what the actual delivery and financing of health care looks like, and how the country that looks most similar to Canada in many respects—the United States—ended up with such different outcomes. In doing so, it is my hope that this book can paint a balanced picture of health care in Canada—the necessary precursor to making sure that we "think the future" in the best possible way.

Why Health Care is Important to Canadians

On the first day of any Canadian politics class, I usually ask my students what, for them, makes Canada "unique." You can imagine the variety of responses I have received over the years, especially at McGill University, where students hail from all points on the map, across Canada and well beyond our borders. Still, the most frequent items the students come back to, time and again, are a variation on the three "H's": (Tim) Hortons, hockey, and health care. The latter shows how profoundly attached many young people feel toward their health care system, but more particularly the kinds of values it embodies and reflects.

Times have changed. Donuts are now a no-no for a new health-conscious generation. Even though hockey retains a strong pull for Canadians, controversy over violence and drawn-out contract disputes have turned plenty of young people off the sport. And as for health care, years of public angst, spending scenarios, and the spectre of the boomer bust have made many young Canadians skittish and scared about the prospects for the future. Students are keener than ever to understand health care as a political issue and policy area, but they are less likely today to find in the Canadian health care "model" a sense of belonging or a national cause. Instead, they are concerned—about its organization, about the costs, and about the future scenarios with which they will be faced.

They are not alone. The parents of my current generation of students might also agree with these views. While Canadians on the whole still support the idea of publicly funded, universal health care, in recent years they have become more concerned about the access to care, and about the associated costs of the system. They are aware of changing demographics, risings costs of new treatments and technology, and changes to funding. These shifts in concerns have been well documented in public opinion polls. Unlike the pundits and pollsters who hang on to every number, how-ever, the academic literature shows that, on things that matter to people, opinion tends to be relatively—and remarkably—stable over time (Page and Shapiro 1992). And health care is arguably one of the most important priorities for Canadians. Which means that, as trends emerge that show changes in public support, it can be big news.

The trends over time do point to rising concern among Canadians about health care as a whole, and dissatisfaction with specific features of their system as well. Since the 1990s, more Canadians have used the word *crisis* to describe health care than ever before. In 1999, for example, an Angus Reid poll suggested that three out of four Canadians (76 percent) felt that the system was in crisis (Vail 2001). Even more telling is the data from comparative public opinion surveys, which have measured notable changes: from a sense of consensus in the 1980s, to a growing discon-tent among Canadians about their health care system through the 1990s (Blendon et al. 1990; Donelan et al. 1999). As we shall see, many of the changes related to health care funding—and the squeeze in delivery of ser-vices—happened during this time period, which may explain part of the trend line (Abelson et al. 2004).

A majority of Canadians do still agree with the values underpinning Canada's health care system (Mendelsohn 2002). And access-to-care sur-veys also show that most Canadians who have contact with the health care system are generally satisfied with the services they receive. Still, uncer-tainty about the system as a whole and uneasiness over sustainability per-sists, revealing a definite erosion in the public's confidence in the future of health care in Canada and, in some cases, more of an openness to alterna-tives to the public system than there has been in the past (Maioni and Martin 2004; Soroka, Maioni and Martin 2013).

This book is an attempt to frame these uncertainties, and hopefully address some of these questions. We know that health care is highly valued by Canadians, but many of us feel like we don't know what the future holds. How can we begin to unpack these concerns?

Citizenship and Health

Canadians' long-standing connection to health care is perhaps best under-stood through the way that social programs came to embody "social citizen-ship" in the post–World War II era (Jenson 1997). We tend to forget that, at the outset, the quest for publicly funded health insurance was part of the larger development of modern welfare states and the extension of social protection across Canada and elsewhere. As such, health care was seen as a part of a wider basket of social policies; it is only in recent decades that health care has become surgically removed from other social provisions in government organizations, and increasingly isolated as a cost-driver that threatens other social programs.

The link between citizenship and social policy has its origins in early 20th century British political thought. One of the best known of these early thinkers is T.H. Marshall, whose conception of the full rights of citizenship included not only civil and political rights, but social rights as well (Marshall 1950). This premise was also part of the influence of another Briton, Sir William Beveridge, who was tasked with developing a postwar reconstruction strategy in the early 1940s. His report had at its core the notion of contributory insurance to ensure a "social minimum" for all citizens. This idea took hold across the Atlantic, too. Lord Beveridge's former student, Leonard Marsh, was the author of Canada's reconstruction report (which has come to be known as the Marsh Report) that recommended nothing less than the implementation of a "social security" state including a federal health care program (Marsh 1975). This blueprint for postwar social security never saw the light of day, since the Liberal government of the time was not receptive to its sweeping proposals; nor, as it turned out, were the provinces, in particular Ontario and Quebec. Still, these foundations eventually became, at least in part, the pillars of the social architecture of the welfare state in Canada. Ironically, even though health care has become one of the most powerful links (if not *the* most powerful) between citizens and their government, between social provision and the notion of Canadian identity, it was not the federal government that designed or innovated the health care systems that are in place today.

Speaking of social rights and citizenship, do we actually have a "right" to health care in Canada? The United Nations' (UN) Universal Declaration of Human Rights includes the right to health, just as the World Health Organization (WHO) refers to the right to the highest attainable standard of health as a "fundamental human right" (Backman et al. 2008, 2047). Canada is a signatory to these treaties, and most Canadians would agree with them, being in the enviable position of having access to health care. Interestingly enough, Canada has had an active role in shaping this international vision, from the participation of John Humphrey in drafting the UN declaration in 1946, to the hosting of the WHO's Ottawa Charter for Health Promotion in 1986.

And yet, health care is not a specific legal "right" protected by the Constitution or the Charter of Rights and Freedoms (although, as we shall see, health-related rights redresses are percolating through the Canadian courts) (Flood and Chen 2010). Relatively few industrialized countries encompass a formal right to health care in their national constitutions, however, although member states of the European Union are now bound by a Charter of Fundamental Rights that includes the right to preventive health care and to medical treatment "under the conditions established by national laws and practices" (European Union 2000, 16).

So, even though rights are not constitutionally enshrined, Canadians do, in practice, enjoy considerably secure access to health and health care in the context of a wider notion of "social security" through the welfare state. But health care differs from other social programs funded by governments in Canada in several ways. Unlike social assistance or employment insurance, or even postsecondary education, it is a pretty sure bet that every single Canadian, at some point in their lives, will need health or medical services and have contact with the health sector in their province. And when they do, it is likely to be in a very personal way, exemplified in the notion of a "care" relationship with health professionals or in a health care establishment. Often, this happens when people are at their most vulnerable (as in an emergency situation), or may well coincide with a joyous occasion (such as the birth of a child) or an extremely difficult experience (a terminal diagnosis or death of a loved one).

Another crucial difference is that government intervention in the health care sector implies a form of rationing of scarce—and expensive—resources. Health care is not a typical consumer good: the basic "demand" for health care is conditioned by need, not want; the demand is mediated by asymmetry of information in which the consumer relies on professional diagnosis; the need is often unpredictable and its cost is usually beyond the capacity of the average individual to pay all at once. In other words, the cost-supply relationship is not that of a typical consumer good. After all, who can really put a price on health?

Of course, this leads to a different set of problems about the definition and scope of what Canadians expect their health care system to deliver and at what cost. In the past generation, the health sector as a whole has been buffeted in paradoxical fashion—on the one hand, by a shift toward prevention of disease and promotion of health, and on the other, the incredible technological breakthroughs in biotech, pharmacology, and intervention procedures. At the same time, a "consumer revolution" is in play, in which the public has become more savvy—and demanding—through the use of digital information to self-diagnose, compare and contrast care alternatives, and demand increasing quantity and quality of care (Decter 2000). And all of this is happening in the context of an acute squeeze on government finances, as calls for lower taxes and constraints on social spending come up against increased expectations and rising costs in the health care sector. Furthermore, as we shall see, there is a larger debate at play about the definition of access to care that involves timeliness, quality, and the notion of a "medical home."

Canada is not alone in relying on public authorities to regulate access to services and redistribute the costs of paying for health care. Almost every industrialized country does so, for part or all of their populations. In Germany and Japan, employees and employers both pay into insurance funds, and then regulate physician fees and hospital prices; UK residents must register with general practitioners, who in turn refer them onward to more specialized forms of care; even the US requires workers to earmark a specific part of their income toward social security taxes for Medicare and to contribute to Medicaid through general taxes.

The Canadian way is to compel residents in the provinces and territories to contribute as taxpayers, and in return guarantee access to care through the publicly funded systems that administer the insurance plan and reimburse the costs of care. Governments also regulate the health care sector, by negotiating fees for services and by imposing certain rules on providers. For this kind of an arrangement to work, there has to be consensus on the role of the state, the relationship between governments and providers of care, and the mutual rights and responsibilities of citizens. It also means that politics very much matter in the health care sector in Canada.

The Politics of Health Care

The classic definition of politics as *who gets what, when, and how* (Lasswell 1936) serves as a basic roadmap of health policy and politics. Governments have an important role to play in deciding how Canadians access and pay for health care, when that care is made available, and how the system itself is organized and financed.

All of these decisions are rife with potential controversy, because they involve money, interests, and power, a heady combination indeed. For example, decisions about money—how much to tax people, and what to do with the monies raised—are at the heart of what governments do in Canada. Public spending on health care has grown over time and now occupies a significant part of provincial budgets. This is an enormous responsibility and one that places a considerable strain on public treasuries, leading to the current debate about whether or not governments can sustain the costs of health care.

Still, at the end of the day, health care services aren't free: they have to be paid for, whether by public plans, private insurance, or individuals paying out of pocket. There is no consensus, either academic or popular, that one of these ways is more sustainable than the other. In fact, we know that public plans tend to contain costs better than the alternatives, although the way they do so—redistribution and rationing—may not always be popular. Part of cost containment also involves deciding on the price of health care.

In public systems across Canada, that price is determined by how much physicians are reimbursed, how hospitals are funded, and how items such as equipment, technology, and pharmaceuticals are paid for.

This is where interests come into play. Medical interests have long been at the heart of political conflict about health care, since the economic livelihood and professional autonomy of the providers are at stake. The development of health insurance in Canada involved several confrontations between physicians and the state, an experience repeated in many other countries with well-developed health care delivery systems and powerful interest groups. In Canada, the compromise that allowed physicians to retain their private practice while agreeing to public payment is one of the unique hallmarks of the system (Naylor 1986), although it too has come under strain.

Some physicians are now seeking to revisit that compromise, to allow more private payment, particularly in diagnostic testing and elective surgery, upsetting the fine balance between cost and access in the delivery of health care. And as physician incomes rise, so too does the scrutiny over fees and modes of reimbursement. More recently, as the cost of drugs has increased, pharmaceutical interests have also come under scrutiny. This is a sector that involves huge political stakes, such as patent laws, drug approval, formulary inclusions, as well as infrastructure development, research investment, and job creation.

With such enormous fiscal stakes and well-organized interests at hand, health care has become an arena of high-stakes power politics. But perhaps the most enduring feature of these politics has to do with the way health care intersects with federal-provincial relations and the institution of federalism itself. Even though health care is a provincial responsibility, the symbolic link between Canada—outside of Quebec—and health care is a strong one. By the same token, health care has come to represent a defining element of Canadian federalism itself, and is often an aspect of intergovernmental affairs that is fraught with tensions.

Federalism is a complicated subject at the best of times, and not all federal systems work the same way. In theory, federalism involves the division of power and the allocation of decision-making among more than one level of government, although this arrangement can vary from "watertight compartments" to more "coordinate" or shared systems (Wheare 1951). In Canada, power is formally divided between the federal government and the provinces, but in many important policy sectors, both levels of government are responsible for insuring the well-being of citizens. Furthermore, Canadian federalism has not been static over time; scholars have been wont to refer to the different "faces" of federalism (Mallory 1965) or the "pendulum" shifts between conflict and co-operation in intergovernmental affairs (Simeon and Robinson 1990).

Much of the literature on comparative welfare states points to the problematic effects of federalism on social policy development (Huber, Ragin, Stephens 1993). There are many examples of the problems that arise when federalism interacts with social policy. First and foremost is the challenge of assigning and identifying jurisdiction in legal or constitutional documents, and then the work of interpreting and operationalizing the roles and responsibilities of each level of power. This often delays or can even preclude coherent policy responses from emerging. Canadian governments' responses to the Great Depression fell into that trap, as did the attempts to build a program of postwar social security. And the constitutional conflicts that marked the federal-provincial relationship in the 1970s, 1980s, and beyond were often preoccupied with refining decision-making powers and cost-sharing, including social policy.

In the American context, federalism and social policy have often fed into the problems of competition between states that can lead to a "race to the bottom" in funding social programs, which may not lead to the best policy outcomes, as the history of social welfare has shown. Furthermore, in an era of fiscal retrenchment, this can also lead to calculations by politicians to engage in "blame avoidance" for difficult policy decisions, which is obviously easier to do in a federal setting (Weaver 1986). In Canada, we have plenty of exposure to this in the health care arena, characterized by a great deal of "long-distance hollering," as former Saskatchewan premier Roy Romanow put it (Commission 2002, 5).

In spite of these problems, federalism can also be thought of as providing a laboratory for subnational experimentation. In this optic, decentralized political systems allow for innovation and policy learning. And the Canadian experience shows that federalism can indeed have a dynamic impact in policy development (Tuohy 1992).

One example of this is how high-level negotiations between the federal government and the provinces led to the Canada Pension Plan (CPP) model and its Quebec counterpart, the Quebec Pension Plan (QPP) (Simeon 1972). The case of health care offers another powerful demonstration of provincial innovation, through Saskatchewan's efforts in setting up North America's first public hospital and medical insurance programs. This also provides an example of policy learning, as the public model was diffused to other provinces through federal spending power.

The development of this particular model of public health insurance in Canada also reveals how political ideas are a crucial factor in the politics of health care.

Comparative scholars often typecast Canada as a "liberal" welfare state, based on a more limited role of government than its European counterparts, and geared toward market exigencies and reinforcing differences in wealth and status rather than embracing a redistributive function (Esping-Andersen 1989). But Canadian scholars have pointed out that Canada is not a "pure" liberal welfare state (Thérien and Noël 1994). This is particularly evident when seen against a North American backdrop, since social programs developed in a much more comprehensive fashion than in the United States.

The design of publicly funded health care in Canada bears this out, since the allocation of services is indeed regulated as a "public good," and governments, both provincial and federal, have a role to play in ensuring that this good is available to all Canadians.

Canada's "imperfect" liberalism has been the stuff of many scholarly debates, including those dealing with the historical origins of a "counter-revolution" against American liberalism (Lipset 1988). Putting aside the spectacle of Loyalists finding a British North America haven, a greater variety of ideas and social forces have indeed found expression in Canadian politics than in the American counterpart, in particular Toryism and socialism (Horowitz 1966).

The impact of Toryism on the Canadian welfare state can be seen in an emphasis on the collective's responsibility to ensure the well-being of the less fortunate in society, rooted deep within the noblesse oblige of the traditional conservative world view. And one can certainly find social-democratic elements, namely equality and solidarity, in the way that health care is financed through general tax revenues, and in the fact that the delivery of health services is predicated on the basis of need rather than the ability to pay.

Outline of the Book

Like its introduction, this book is designed to help understand the importance of health care in Canada, and how the development of such an important policy domain helps us understand even more about Canada as a whole. And, just as these first pages have covered a lot of ground, so too does the rest of the book, as it attempts to take a broad lens to the study of health care: historical, descriptive, comparative. The focus throughout is to explain and contextualize the considerable challenges that we face in making decisions about the future of health care in Canada.

Chapter 1 starts at the beginning and looks at the historical origins and the specific political and societal forces that shaped health care development over time in Canada. Chapters 2 and 3 take on the task of describing and explaining the landscape of health care organization and financing in Canada, and attempt to bring clarity to the complex details that govern how we receive and pay for health care. In Chapters 4 and 5, the Canadian experience is situated against the backdrop of the experiences of other industrialized countries, a comparison that includes our closest neighbour, the United States, and two European models from the UK and Germany. Chapter 6 offers a glimpse into the essential but often-overlooked wealth and diversity of experience across the provinces, with a focus on the distinctive features that shaped health care systems in Saskatchewan and Quebec.

Finally, Chapter 7 turns back to some of the lessons learned from this journey through health care development, financing, and organization, and suggests a roadmap for understanding future directions.

Chapter 1

The History of Health Care in Canada

Canadians like to think of themselves as innovators in social policy, having developed a safety net for citizens that includes publicly funded health insurance from coast to coast, and lauding such "great" Canadians as Tommy Douglas, the "founder" of medicare. But the historical record is far from a picture-perfect postcard. Instead, it reveals a hard-fought political battle that was far from a foregone conclusion at the outset and whose outcomes were unpredictable.

What Tommy Douglas knew, and what many Canadians working in cities or rural areas shared, was the experience of living through decades of brutal economic circumstances. In these conditions, life was tough, and new ideas and political movements—born of despair at the existing political situation, and hope for a better collective future—had ample room to grow and spread. It is from these roots that the historical development of health insurance in Canada takes its form.

The Long Road to . . . No Health Insurance

For all of Wilfrid Laurier's boast that the 20th century would belong to Canada, in the early 1900s it was a far from idyllic place to live, particularly for new immigrants, homesteaders, and low-wage workers in urban environments. Apart from quarantine and the most basic of public health concerns under the responsibility of the federal government, and provincial regulation of hospitals and charitable institutions as stipulated in the British North America Act of 1867, health care was not considered part of the public realm. Instead, family, community, and church were the main sources of succour for the ill or infirm and, increasingly, municipal services that offered relief for the medically indigent. As the population of the country grew, and urbanization increased, these kinds of comforts became less and less certain for more and more people.

While liberalism stretched to embrace social reform in Britain, leading to a new system of state medicine in 1911 (see Chapter 5), and the progressive movement endorsed a similar model in the US in 1912 (see Chapter 4), in Canada it was not until after World War I that reformist ideals entered the political discourse. It was a tumultuous time, as labour unions became more militant in their quest for better working conditions and wages. This militancy often took place alongside more socialist efforts, leading to the kinds of confrontation—a good example is the Winnipeg General Strike in 1919—that were a harbinger of new, radical ideas in Canada. Added to this was the emergence of farmer-based third parties in Ontario and the west, attempting to make their voices heard in provincial legislatures. In Alberta, the United Farmers government was publicly committed to "state medicine"; in neighbouring Saskatchewan, rural hospital districts were created, allowing for municipal taxes to retain doctors.

But the notion of social insurance as a basis for government action had not taken hold on the Canadian political scene. The federal Liberal Party was the first major Canadian political party to endorse social insurance. In 1919, after choosing William Lyon Mackenzie King as leader, the party adopted a new platform that included federal-provincial action toward "an adequate system of insurance against unemployment, sickness and dependence in old age" (Bryden 1974, 66). Also in 1919, a Dominion Department of Health was established, designed mainly to coordinate federal activities in public health. This was particularly important in light of the epidemics of influenza and the plight of returning soldiers that characterized the immediate postwar period.

King had previously played an important role in developing labour policy as the Department of Labour's first deputy minister. In 1918, he published *Industry and Humanity*, a treatise that heralded the need for a larger role for the state in the economy, including the social arena. But by the time he became prime minister in 1921, King's primary concern was trying to maintain power in light of a significant political opposition made up of the farmer-dominated Progressive Party and Labour independents in the House of Commons. In an increasingly tense political climate—which would culminate in a constitutional crisis—labour MPs J.S. Woodsworth and A.A. Heaps of Winnipeg were pivotal in precipitating the passage of old age pensions legislation just before the 1926 election. Surviving *in extremis*, the Liberal government set up a Select Standing Committee on Industrial and International Relations to examine unemployment, invalidity, and sickness insurance (including a "national health programme"). Its report recommended that the provinces initiate any legislative action, given their constitutional jurisdiction, although the federal government could provide grants along the lines of the new old age pensions system (Guest 1980).

With these constitutional caveats as a backdrop, and given King's penchant for fiscal restraint, the onset of the Great Depression was unlikely to compel him to act boldly in the area of health or social insurance. His government's inaction, however, was met with loud criticism. Goaded by questions from J.S. Woodsworth and other Labour members in the House of Commons on the government's insufficient unemployment and relief efforts, King lashed out against the provincial governments' demands for monies for "alleged unemployment purposes" and declared, "I would not give them a five-cent piece" (Bothwell, Drummond, and English 1987, 260). This "Five-Cent Speech," one of King's rare political mistakes, cost him the 1930 election, and also contributed to the Liberal Party's loss of credibility as the party of social reform.

The link that Roosevelt's New Deal made in the United States between economic and social renewal was not an idea shared by many political leaders in Canada, and certainly not Mackenzie King. In fact, Canada's New Deal was not a Liberal initiative, but rather one designed by Conservative Prime Minister R.B. Bennett. The Conservative government's initial response to the Depression was limited, through public work relief and higher tariffs, although Bennett was later forced to resort to more urgent measures, such as setting up work camps for single unemployed men in 1931, and implementing direct relief in 1932 (Neatby 1972).

The pressure on government came also from professional associations. Canadian physicians felt the effects of the Depression keenly, as even middle-class families found it more and more difficult to pay medical fees. In addition, the indigent medical care system financed through municipalities and charitable works was unable to meet the increased demand. Although unpaid service was already a problem for doctors in the 1920s, it reached crisis proportions in the 1930s. The Canadian Medical Association (CMA) attempted to push governments to set up medical relief to alleviate the financial burden of non-remunerated care. The most drastic action came in Manitoba, where physicians in Winnipeg temporarily withdrew all but emergency services to relief recipients to protest the absence of a medical relief policy that would offer payment to doctors (Bothwell and English 1981).

As the federal Conservatives fell out of public favour, their provincial counterparts had fallen in British Columbia, Saskatchewan, Nova Scotia, and Ontario. The party was losing support not only to the Liberals but also to third-party protest movements throughout the prairie provinces in areas of traditional Conservative strength.

Facing an election in 1935, Bennett finally turned to the social insurance platform, inspired by reform measures in the US and in Britain. During a visit to London for an Imperial Conference in 1933, Bennett met with the British minister of labour to discuss unemployment and health insurance, and on returning gave instructions to begin studying similar types of proposals for Canada. In November 1934, the Canadian government authorized senior civil servants to travel to Washington for Roosevelt's National Conference on Economic Security (Struthers 1983).

The Bennett "New Deal" for Canada was unveiled in January 1935, proclaiming a commitment to "social justice" and promising government action on minimum wages and working hours, unemployment insurance, farm support, a new old age pensions program—and even health insurance. It was a surprise to most Canadians, including the Conservative caucus and most of the cabinet. The Employment and Social Insurance Act (ESI) that derived from Bennett's New Deal was not a radical program, except insofar as it treaded on provincial jurisdiction. The health provisions were exceptionally vague, pledging federal co-operation for collecting health insurance data and information, and stipulating the review of any proposed scheme with the provinces, municipalities, or private groups.

Although the ESI Act passed, its implementation was delayed by the federal election in the fall of 1935. With a platform that declared "King or Chaos," the Liberal Party won over 70 percent of the seats in the House of Commons. King referred the ESI Act to the Privy Council for judicial review, where its provisions, including those concerning health matters, were judged ultra vires in 1937. Rather than launch his own New Deal, King instead appointed a Royal Commission to investigate jurisdictional and fiscal conflicts that had rendered the ESI Act ineffective.

While the federal government may have dithered on health and social insurance during the Great Depression, it was a topic of considerable concern in the provinces—and it was in British Columbia that the question of health insurance would become most significant. As early as 1919, a Royal Commission on State Health Insurance was appointed, but its recommendations for a system of health insurance were not implemented; instead, the legislature passed a resolution urging federal action on the matter in 1922. By the time a second Royal Commission reported in 1932, the pressure for legislative action in health insurance had been heightened by the impact of the Great Depression. This report advocated compulsory insurance for lower-income workers, with voluntary participation for all other residents, and the Liberal premier, Thomas "Duff" Pattullo, was committed to implementing these recommendations (Fisher 1991). In British Columbia—a province that had developed the most radical blend of protest politics and labour militancy in Canada, and facing a left-wing opposition—Pattullo may also have been encouraged to take this stand out of political necessity.

While the public was generally in favour of health insurance, there was a clear split over the issue: Labour, the left, progressive Liberals, and lower-income workers against business, organized medicine, and conservative Liberals. In addition, although Pattullo tried to convince King that increased public spending was the only way to rid the Liberal Party of the threat from the left, the prime minister refused to commit to any financial guarantees. Business interests were concerned about the contributions required by employers to finance health insurance, and feared higher taxes associated with the health plan would give eastern competitors a market advantage.

Doctors participated in the drafting of the initial legislation, and supported the government's plan because it covered the indigent and limited compulsory insurance to low-wage earners. This meant that BC doctors, reeling from the economic impact of the Depression themselves, could be assured payment from higher-risk economic groups. In addition, they could finally count on compensation for the unpaid care they were expected to provide in some measure to the less fortunate. But serious financial constraints, including the federal refusal to guarantee funds and business opposition to higher taxes, forced the Pattullo government to modify the plan, notably by eliminating indigent coverage. With a prime economic incentive removed from the plan, doctors began to express reservations about the rest of the arrangement, particularly the sweeping powers of the proposed BC Health Commission and the "state control" over the autonomy of physicians and their fees inherent in the plan (Naylor 1986).

The BC government finally passed the health insurance bill in early 1936, but the plan's implementation was postponed until the next provincial election in June 1937. This election coincided with a referendum that found 59 percent of British Columbians supported comprehensive health insurance. Borrowing a useful tactic from Prime Minister King, Pattullo suspended further action on health insurance until the report of the Royal Commission that had been appointed to study federal-provincial relations. By the end of the decade, as the BC Liberal Party settled in for a second term, its most prominent reform package—health insurance—was shelved indefinitely.

War and the Postwar Welfare State

War and health have always been related, as many breakthroughs in medical care were born on the battlefield. But in the Canadian experience, it was the impact of war on the home front that had important consequences in the 1940s. The heightened debates over postwar social security and the rise in support for voices from the left, in Ottawa and the provinces, changed the discourse of social reform and laid the path for health policy.

The first order of business was to figure out who exactly had a say on health and social matters. The 1940 report of the Royal Commission on Dominion-Provincial Relations (the Rowell-Sirois Report) agreed that health insurance was a provincial matter, but suggested that the federal government had a role to play through its fiscal spending power. This set off considerable bureaucratic interest within the Department of Pensions and National Health, through the minister, Ian Mackenzie, and his senior civil servant, J.J. Heagerty, a public health doctor who was well versed in the history of medicine and convinced of the inevitability of health insurance. By 1941, Heagerty's team had drafted three model bills on health insurance (provincial plan, federal plan via constitutional amendment, and an enabling act for the provinces). Although Mackenzie tried to convince the prime minister of the importance of health insurance as part of post-war reconstruction, King balked at the financial implications. Nevertheless, he did agree to set up an interdepartmental Advisory Committee on Health Insurance (Taylor 1987).

By December 1942, the advisory council's revised draft bills were completed, one an enabling act authorizing federal contributions to provincially administered health insurance plans, the other a model bill for the provinces.

But as the cabinet was still divided, King compromised by appointing a Special Committee on Social Security to review the proposals for the House of Commons.

The 1943 hearings occurred in an atmosphere charged by the visit of Lord Beveridge, the architect of Britain's postwar reconstruction plan, and the release of the report of the Canadian Advisory Committee on Reconstruction (Marsh 1975). Although the committee was chaired by the principal of McGill University, Cyril James, its report would be remembered for its author, Leonard Marsh, a former member of the League for Social Reconstruction (the brain trust of the left-wing Co-operative Commonwealth Federation, or CCF). While federal bureaucrats favoured administration by the provinces, Marsh recommended a federal health insurance plan via constitutional amendment (similar to unemployment insurance in 1940).

By this time, the medical community was concerned that a health care plan might be developed without their approval. Having endorsed the principle of health insurance, the Canadian Medical Association attempted to contribute to the bureaucratic proposals, including suggestions of fee-for-service payment and indigent coverage. But the political concern was that the plan not turn into a "doctor's bill," which would be hard to sell to working Canadians.

Nervous about opposition from the left, especially over social reform, the Liberal government's 1944 Throne Speech emphasized social security, including health insurance, as a key feature of postwar reconstruction, after negotiations with the provinces. And the provincial scene changed irrevocably that year when the CCF won its first contest in Saskatchewan in an election fought on the health insurance issue.

Despite the political attractiveness of health care, the Liberal government—and especially the cautious King—was as wary as always of the twin dragons of jurisdiction and money, so, the fate of health care was tied to the larger postwar agenda and a new fiscal federalism. King lost his own seat in the CCF sweep of Saskatchewan in 1945, but his party squeaked to a majority—having stressed the link between "Liberalism and Labour." The ensuing Dominion-Provincial conference would be the test, but the conference ended in deadlock with a lack of consensus on the revenue arrangements and taxation control.

Paul Martin Sr., the new minister of national health and welfare, proposed a compromise solution to Prime Minister King: the Liberal government could "keep faith" on its promises by inaugurating more modest reform through a program of national health grants to the provinces. Part of the larger bureaucratic blueprint for health reform, this initiative would provide federal grants-in-aid for public health measures and hospital construction in the provinces. Not all of the Liberal cabinet agreed with Martin's assertion that this was the first step in the "ultimate goal" of health insurance, but it certainly helped the government save face on the issue. The provinces, and even the medical lobby, were also in accord, and the plan was implemented in 1948.

Provincial Innovation, Federal Cost-Sharing

The health grants program would prove to be especially important for Saskatchewan. A rural, economically challenged province in mid-century, Saskatchewan's need for health infrastructure was acute, particularly in the context of the promises that had been made by the new CCF government. The decision to begin with hospital insurance, passed in 1946 and implemented in 1947, avoided the direct confrontation with physicians that had plagued British Columbia's earlier efforts and coordinated with existing rural hospital plans. It also set the path for public financing of hospitals that remained voluntary institutions, which would be become the norm across the Canadian provinces, rather than having them become nationalized, as would be the case with the National Health Service (NHS) in Britain.

While expensive for the public treasury, the hospital plan turned out to be a popular success and within only a few years, copycat legislation was in place in British Columbia and Alberta (although funding mechanisms differed there). Still, it bothered Premier Tommy Douglas that his province had been forced to "go it alone" in this expensive undertaking, slowing down efforts to have a full system of "medicare" in place (Taylor 1987, 69). And Douglas was not the only premier pushing the federal government; by the early 1950s, Ontario was also moving toward hospital insurance. Although led by Progressive Conservative Leslie Frost, the Ontario government was under considerable pressure—from the left and the labour movement, but also a wider swathe of public opinion. But Frost, the most practical of politicians, wanted cost-sharing guarantees, and he wanted them from the Liberal government in Ottawa.

Prime Minister Louis St. Laurent was hardly a social reformer; his leanings were toward fiscal prudence and his Quebec roots made him wary of jurisdictional overreach. His position was that there could be no federal plan until provinces signalled they wanted one. Bureaucrats under Minister Paul Martin were busy at work studying the matter, and most agreed that Saskatchewan's successful precedent with hospital insurance could become the model for a federal cost-sharing program. In the House of Commons, the CCF—with the feisty Stanley Knowles leading the charge—exhorted the government to make good on its electoral promises. The right-wing Social Credit Party rejected the whole idea as "socialized medicine," while the Progressive Conservatives mocked the CCF's "obsession" with health insurance. But Martin would also make good use of the CCF threat in "convincing the doubters" in the Liberal Party of the political saliency of health reform (Martin 1985).

At the 1955 Federal-Provincial Conference, Ontario and Saskatchewan agreed they were ready; the Social Credit governments of Alberta and British Columbia insisted that any federal grants should be free of conditions; and Quebec and Manitoba wanted to retain full autonomy over health care. In early 1956, the federal government outlined a proposal for hospital and diagnostic services: to share one-half of the operating costs with the provinces, provided that the services were available to all residents, without "excessive" financial deterrents. The plan would also require a double majority before implementation—a majority of provinces, representing a majority of Canadians.

In early 1957, with five provinces, including Ontario, on board, legislation was passed. It was a unanimous vote in the House of Commons— a result that highlighted the issue's political stakes while also undermining its saliency for the Liberal Party in the ensuing election campaign. In June, the Liberal Party's run of 22 years in power came to an end. The new Progressive Conservative minority government removed the majority province rule that fall, enabling federal participation in hospital insurance to begin in July 1958; in March of that year, they reaped the reward of a landslide election victory.

By 1960, nine of the 10 Canadian provinces had introduced hospital insurance programs under the Hospital Insurance and Diagnostic Services Act. Quebec would sign on after the historic defeat of the Union Nationale by the Liberal Party under Jean Lesage, and hospital insurance would become one of the first of many new measures associated with the Quiet Revolution.

A collateral impact of the new cost-sharing program meant that Saskatchewan, perennially squeezed financially, could now focus attention on the unfinished business of the CCF's health reform agenda, namely medical insurance. For Tommy Douglas, under pressure to join the party's federal wing, it promised a fitting finale to his career in provincial politics. In December 1959, Douglas outlined plans for universal medical care based on fee-for-service reimbursement, the basis of the pilot project that had been tested in Swift Current in 1946 and, it was thought, a more palatable option for the medical profession.

However, there was little love lost between the CCF government and the medical profession, represented by the Saskatchewan College of Physicians and Surgeons (SCPS). In addition to concerns about professional autonomy, there was also at stake the future of the rapidly growing and lucrative profession-sponsored medical insurance plans. So, the 1960 election galvanized physician opposition and saw the launch of a widespread public relations campaign against "socialized medicine." The election became a referendum on the government's plan for medical insurance, which the CCF won.

In this highly charged atmosphere, even the Canadian Medical Association lobbied the federal government to defuse the situation. Prime Minister John Diefenbaker responded by setting up a Royal Commission on health services and financing, led by Saskatchewan's chief justice, Emmett Hall. The CMA hoped this would bolster confidence in the private delivery of medical services, while at the same time defuse demands for public medical insurance.

The only way doctors could accept medical insurance, it was argued, was if the profession had autonomy in administering the plan and controlling the method of payment. Obviously, this was not acceptable to the Saskatchewan government. Their legislation was duly passed in November, but its implementation was stalled by the SCPS's refusal to negotiate with the newly created Medical Care Insurance Commission.

In May 1962, the SCPS called a special meeting and prepared for strike action. That June, Tommy Douglas led the recently formed New Democratic Party (the former CCF) to an abysmal showing in his first foray into federal politics, with the medical lobby, business interests, and the highly vocal "Keep Our Doctors" committees active throughout Saskatchewan. On July 1, 1962, the start date for implementation, doctors in the province withdrew all but emergency services.

Despite the support of the CMA, the Saskatchewan doctors' strike action became a public relations disaster, with loud criticism of the ethics and legality of their actions. After three weeks, aware of rising public resentment, the SCPS agreed to mediation. The doctors accepted the extra-billing concessions proposed by the government and won the right to maintain profession-sponsored voluntary plans.

The Saskatchewan conflict had an immediate and lasting impact on the wider debate over medical insurance in Canada. The confrontation riveted public opinion and propelled medical insurance onto the national political agenda. For some, the use of strike action by physicians crossed a line that would reduce the medical profession's prestige and influence, with their opposition to reform associated with self-interest rather than the concerns of their patients and public. Even though it would not be last time that physicians would resort to strike action, the overwhelmingly negative public reaction may have convinced the CMA to back off that possibility in the ensuing debate with the federal government.

The report of the Hall Commission (the Royal Commission on Health Services) reflected this weakening of the medical lobby. Released in 1964, the report rejected the CMA's proposals for voluntary medical insurance (already under consideration in Alberta and Ontario) and means-tested subsidies in favour of federal cost-sharing toward "comprehensive, universal, provincial programs of personal health services" (MacDermot 1967, 89). In the original report, these included not only medical care but also drug, prosthetic, and home care for all, and dental and optical services for specific groups. It was a breathtaking sweep of recommendations that, for the first time, articulated a set of fundamental principles about the role of the individual and the state in health matters, embodied in a "Health Charter for Canadians."

By the time the Hall Report was released, the Liberal Party was back in power, with a new leader, Lester Pearson, and a new progressive program. Universal health insurance was a main plank in the platform designed to co-opt potential NDP supporters. And, in the House of Commons, the Liberal minority government had to contend with the NDP as a third party pushing the health insurance agenda. The Hall Report's recommendations became an important focus for "progressive" Liberals, in opposition to the old guard of the party, and the business and medical communities.

The Liberal government was also concerned about the potential for a crazy quilt of medical insurance plans to emerge in the provinces, anathema to their vision for harmonized fiscal and social policy. At the July 1965 Federal-Provincial Conference, Prime Minister Pearson unveiled the necessary criteria that provincial medicare plans would have to meet for federal funding. These principles included: public administration of provincial medical plans; comprehensive benefits, with generalist and specialist services as the "initial minimum"; the portability of these benefits for all Canadians as they travelled from province to province; and universality, so that all provincial residents would be covered "on uniform terms and conditions." The ensuing election campaign promised medical insurance across Canada by the centennial year, July 1967, but rifts within the Liberal government on the issue continued. Even though the bill and passage occurred in 1966, it would take two more years to implement the cost-sharing plan.

How the provinces implemented medical insurance is a fascinating history in and of itself. By 1968, only two provinces (Saskatchewan and British Columbia) had pre-existing medical plans that could be easily adapted to the federal government cost-sharing plan. In Alberta, where Social Credit Premier Ernest Manning had led a campaign against "socialistic" health insurance in favour of voluntary "Manningcare," the plan had a profound impact on federal-provincial relations. In Ontario, Progressive Conservative Premier John Robarts made his opposition public. But two things convinced recalcitrant premiers to step in line with the federal plan: first was the undeniable pressure of public opinion (there was growing public demand), and second was the obvious loss of federal funds being made available (funded through a 2 percent federal tax hike had been imposed to ensure financial viability).

Quebec provides perhaps the most interesting story (see Chapter 6). While the Liberal government of Jean Lesage had implemented hospital insurance in 1961, his government remained critical of federal intrusion in provincial jurisdiction, and had mounted a defence of "opting-out" of federal initiatives with financial compensation in developing Quebec's pension plan. Although this failed to win the day in the case of health care, Quebec took its time in joining the cost-sharing medical plan, and ended up designing a system different from those in other provinces. Two of the main differences were limiting the ability of physicians to opt out, and outlawing extra billing. While general practitioners came on board, specialists remained opposed. Their ill-timed strike in October 1970 ended in defeat—the Quebec government was able to pass emergency measures that put into place the medical insurance law, and forced the specialists back to work.

The following year, the *Loi sur les services de santé et les services sociaux* put into place a distinctive health care system that included "global medicine" as part of an integrated system of health and social services, and the creation of CLSCs (local community service centres), public health departments, and regional health boards. The law was unique in Canada in that it emphasized primary care, made room for the integration of health and social services based on community-centred access, and included the regionalization of services in an explicit attempt to decentralize decision-making.

Changing the Rules of the Game

By 1972, all of the provinces had signed on to the cost-sharing program. Almost immediately, the economic pressures of the 1970s forced the federal government to replace the open-ended cost-sharing with block grants in 1977 through the Established Programs Financing Act for health care and postsecondary education. From that point on, the provinces would be responsible for cost control, since the federal transfers would be calculated on a per capita basis, with increases tied to economic growth rather than the actual cost of health care.

Obviously, considerable federal-provincial tension ensued over who was responsible for ensuring adequate funding of health care. And, as health costs increased, financial pressures opened the door to user fees in some provinces and an increase in extra billing by doctors.

It was to ensure adherence to a form of national standards, and to operationalize the fiscal levers that would lead to this, that the federal government passed the Canada Health Act (CHA) in 1984. It was devised under the leadership of Health Minister Monique Bégin, and would prove to be the last—and arguably one of the most important—policy legacies of Pierre Trudeau's tenure in power. Short, terse, but powerful, the Act spelled out the five principles to which provincial health systems would heretofore need to adhere: universality, comprehensiveness, portability, public administration, and equal access. The latter provision effectively ruled out extra billing and user fees, and threatened the imposition of dollar-for-dollar financial sanctions on the provinces that tolerated such practices.

Several provinces were forced to change their legislation as a consequence, and not without political fireworks. In Ontario, specialists went on strike in 1987 to protest these changes, but they found, as had been the case in Saskatchewan and in Quebec, that this had negative consequences in terms of public opinion (Tuohy 1988).

Despite ensuing federal-provincial tensions, politicians throughout Canada tended to support the public insurance system, since it maintained considerable public support. Even as Brian Mulroney's Progressive Conservative government attempted to reshape elements of the welfare state, health care was left untouched. It would not be exaggerated to claim that health care was—for the latter decades of the 20th century—the most popular social program across Canada.

Things began to change in the 1990s, as a stark economic climate and sharply reduced federal transfers put considerable financial pressure on the provinces, leading to rapidly implemented hospital closures, freezes or caps on the fees charged by health care professionals, and reductions to medical school admissions. Provincial governments coped as best they could, but felt the backlash from public-sector workers in health-related areas, health care professionals, and the public. Despite the salience of health care as an electoral issue, and the Liberal government's strategic use of health care as a wedge issue against its opponents, erosion in public confidence was beginning to emerge.

Prime Minister Jean Chrétien used the situation to his advantage. He appointed former Saskatchewan NDP Premier Roy Romanow to head a Commission on the Future of Health Care in Canada, and by the time it reported in 2002, a more positive economic climate was allowing the federal government to loosen its purse strings. The Romanow Report, as it came to be known, outlined some of the key funding needs in health care; highlighted areas in need of reform (such as primary care and home care); and issued a call to study a national pharmacare strategy. Meanwhile, a report from the Senate Standing Committee on Social Affairs, led by a dynamic Liberal senator, Michael Kirby, was published the same year, and focused attention on wait times for services, underscoring that access to care could be compromised by barriers beyond the financial. In 2005, a Supreme Court case that struck down elements of Quebec's health care laws came to a similar conclusion.

The political response to this mounting public frustration and provincial pressure was unfolding. A new Liberal prime minister, Paul Martin Jr., was at the helm. Despite his past experience as the finance minister responsible for significant cuts to health and social transfers in 1995, Martin seemed intent on re-engaging the provinces in a new kind of collaborative federalism, especially as federal coffers were in a surplus situation. This came to the fore in 2004, as he convened the provincial premiers to a high-profile round of talks on health care financing. The result was an historic federal-provincial accord that, for the first time, put in place a 10-year plan that guaranteed health transfers to the provinces with a 6 percent annual increase to help toward the reinvestment in health care. It was a plan crafted to include both specific goals to improve health care organization and delivery (such as primary care reform) and popular promises that were seen as politically valuable for all involved (such as wait time reductions).

Still, as many governments had learned in the past, health care promises do not always translate into immediate electoral gains, and in 2006, the

Liberal government lost the federal election to a newly formed Conservative Party under Stephen Harper. Ironically, it would be this right-wing party—devoted to provincial autonomy, tax reduction, and ostensibly less rather than more government spending—that would become responsible for doling out the billions of extra transfer dollars for health care under Martin's 10-year plan.

Despite the plan in place, the costs of health care continue to place a heavy burden on provincial treasuries, with no lessening of the political stakes surrounding health reform. For the time being, the federal government has taken a back-seat approach to policy activism in the health care sector, focusing its activities on public health and the health of those "classes" of people for whom they have jurisdictional responsibility, such as Aboriginal groups.

While the 10-year accord can be seen as an example of federal-provincial bargaining, or at least dialogue, the next health care funding decisions may point to a different intergovernmental framework. In late 2011, Finance Minister Jim Flaherty declared that the 6 percent annual increase would be extended to 2016, with subsequent funding tied to economic growth (but with a guarantee of at least 3 percent).

If one thinks of Canadian federalism as a pendulum between forces of more centralized policy-making from Ottawa and a more decentralized policy environment with emphasis on the provinces, then the swing currently seems to be in the latter direction. The Council of the Federation, an initiative to flex provincial leadership that began in 2003, is indicative of this shift: an interprovincial institution for discussion and, to some extent, decision-making between the provinces. With the end of federal largesse in sight, the provincial premiers have used this assembly to find a way forward in health care reform. In 2012, two working groups were set up—on innovations in health care, and on fiscal arrangements—in an attempt to address this.

Still, the years ahead loom large as a new chapter in the evolution of health care in Canada, and the delicate dialogue between provincial and federal governments. It may be that the 10-year accord will end with a whimper rather than a bang, as the federal government reiterates its preference for provincial leadership in health care, and provincial governments may be loath to tally up the fits and starts of health reform over the past decade. Nevertheless, it seems clear that the fiscal and organizational challenges of health systems across Canada will continue to dominate provincial politics and shape public preferences for a long time to come.

Chapter 2

A Portrait of Health Care in Canada

Is there really a "Canadian health care system?" The prevailing sentiment is that yes, there is. In fact, this sentiment is so pervasive that not only do Canadians believe this is the case, but even the comparative literature on health care systems routinely refers to Canada in this way.

And yet, health care organization and delivery in Canada is far from a single "system." Instead, it is best envisioned as a mosaic, mixture, or medley of a number of health care systems across the country, with each province and territory responsible for the organization and financing of health care services for its residents.

Indeed, in many ways, health care represents the extensive decentralization that exists in the mix of Canadian social policies. Unlike in other federal polities—such as Germany or Australia—health care in Canada is not a constitutionally shared jurisdiction since it remains in the purview of the provinces. Moreover, the central government does not retain a hands-on role in administration or funding decisions. In fact, even the US federal government has a more active role in health care than its Canadian counterpart, through a direct responsibility for the Medicare program.

The academic literature abounds with examples of the ways in which federalism can help or, in most cases, hinder the development and functioning of welfare states. The difficulties of reaching consensus, the potential for dysfunctional practices of blame avoidance, even the "long-distance hollering" that Roy Romanow has referred to are all parts of the politics of federalism. Be that as it may, the very nature of health care organization and financing in Canada reflects the unique federal landscape of our political system.

And this landscape has come to be dominated by the recurring myth of health care as a core part of Canadian identity and even, in some instances, as a nation-building exercise. Part of the mythmaking has to do with the way in which successive federal governments—in particular, Liberal governments—have worn the mantle of health care to carve out a political space and foster national sentiment around the ideals it represents.

The Division of Powers and Health Care

The men responsible for Confederation had scant interest in the nation involving itself in such personal concerns, hence the absence of the term *health care* in the original British North America Act of 1867. Still, from the division of powers enumerated in that document, responsibilities for health care have become established. Overall, it is the provinces that have primary responsibility for health care, although, constitutionally speaking, the federal government can still choose to play a considerable role (Bräen 2004).

And, as Canadian governments have morphed into their modern states, they have become responsible for a considerable swathe of social protection. Section 92(7) of the Constitution Act of 1982 set out specific powers to provinces. In particular, the act gives provincial legislatures exclusive jurisdiction to enact laws for the "Establishment, Maintenance, and Management of Hospitals, Asylums, Charities and Eleemosynary Institutions." An eleemosynary institution is, in British legal parlance, devoted to the provision of alms and usually refers to places that provide these alms to the poor and sick; these institutions derive from the notion of the "deserving" poor at the heart of poor laws that were influential not only in Britain but across its colonies as well.

From this constitutional provision, provinces draw the ability to legislate in matters related to the regulation and funding of health care establishments. Section 92(13) gives provinces legal authority over "Property and Civil Rights in the Province," and section 92(16) gives them jurisdiction over "Generally all Matters of a merely local or private Nature in the Province." This allows provinces further leeway in regulating and reimbursing health care providers, for example.

The federal government, meanwhile, does have constitutional responsibilities in the wider definitions of health and health care. In 1867, an important concern of public authorities was the spread of disease and the need for adequate quarantine, particularly in the context of immigration, mainly by sea. Thus, it is no surprise that the federal government was accorded a particular responsibility for "quarantine and the establishment and maintenance of marine hospitals" under Section 91(11).

With reference to the general welfare of certain "classes" of people that were considered to have a special relationship with the state, the federal government is also responsible for "Indians" and "aliens"—as they were referred to—as well as inmates of federal penitentiaries and members of the military. Over time, this has expanded to include other Aboriginal peoples, refugees, and veterans.

However, it was the general federal spending power that opened up an important role for the central government to bolster the fiscal capacity of provinces and to facilitate the diffusion of health benefits across the country. This refers to the power the federal government derives from its jurisdiction over "Public Debt and Property" in Section 91(1A) and its taxing power under Section 91(3). The crux of the 1940 Royal Commission on Dominion-Provincial Relations was to zero in on this financial lever, paving the way for a federal role in the development of the postwar Canadian welfare state.

Since 1982, many scholars have interpreted the constitution, and Supreme Court statements, as pointing to a strong rationale for a federal role, such as jurisdiction over criminal law and setting standards through the Canada Health Act (Leeson 2004).

The Canada Health Act

In a postwar era characterized by "co-operative federalism," the federal government was able to deploy its spending power in encouraging the diffusion of a health care model based on the demonstration effect of Saskatchewan's experiments. This was overlaid by explicit notions of the role of the federal government in ensuring core principles that had been an essential feature of the Hall Commission report. For the Liberal governments of the time, this was also a process of grafting "welfare liberalism" onto the party's raison d'être.

The most powerful action in this regard is the Canada Health Act of 1984, which has come to represent the "right" to health care for Canadians, even though this is a far from explicit measure in the legislation.

Passed in the waning days of Pierre Trudeau's last tenure in office, the CHA was ostensibly a measure designed to allow the federal government a means to ensure that the principles already part of the original hospital and medical care legislation would be respected by the provinces (Bégin 1987). The federal government's 1977 decision to change the modus of funding— from cost-sharing to fixed block grants—had put considerable financial pressure on provincial governments, and caused considerable concern about the ways in which additional revenue streams were being tolerated as a result.

As Emmett Hall pointed out once again, when asked to review his Royal Commission report in 1979, allowing the use of extra billing by physicians and moving toward user fees in the provision of care threatened to undermine the basic principles of the existing federal health care legislation. But with block transfers in place, there was little in the fiscal arrangements that would allow the federal government to coherently enforce these conditions, short of withholding the entire cash portion of the grant to a province (Taylor 1987).

The federal response was to design the Canada Health Act, which had two major goals. The first was a practical matter: to give the federal government a fiscal lever to enforce conditions on the money it allocated to the provinces for health care. The act reaffirmed the existing principles of federal legislation (having to do with public administration, universality, portability, and comprehensiveness) and added an additional principle of accessibility. This principle affirmed that health care services must be offered on equal terms and conditions, putting into effect a ban on practices that would allow access to care by other means. The fiscal lever would be the ability of a federal minister of health to identify and call out any province that allowed such practices, and to recommend dollar-for-dollar penalties if they persisted.

The second goal was to carve out a visible and powerful space for the federal government in health care, over and above the fiscal measures at its disposal. In fact, the act amalgamated existing federal cost-sharing legislation—ponderously detailed and relatively obscure for most Canadians—into a short, clear, and highly recognizable "Canada" Health Act, branding the notion of "Canadian" health care onto the public consciousness. While the Canada Health Act was eventually passed by all three major parties in the House of Commons (the Liberal Party, the Progressive Conservative opposition, and the New Democratic Party), the legislation embodied principles crucial to the Liberal government's vision of federalism and national unity.

In a political era in which the federal government was exerting considerable pressure on nation-building—particularly through constitutional reforms and the Charter of Rights and Freedoms—the Canada Health Act became part of a larger perception of the moral leadership the federal government sought to develop in this field.

Through the haze of history, we tend to forget the discontent of provincial reaction to the measure, and the outrage of doctors as well. The provinces argued that they had not been properly consulted and that the act infringed on provincial jurisdiction for health care. This was especially important in Quebec, where the government argued there was no justification to impose federal "norms" since these principles were already expressed in Quebec's own legislation, which represented the real link between state and society in this regard (Maioni 1999).

Doctors, meanwhile, saw the act as an infringement of their freedom, and, in Ontario, became part of wider political unrest during the late 1980s

(Tuohy 1988). As an unwieldy coalition of Ontario Liberals and NDP developed new health care legislation to conform to the Canada Health Act by banning extra billing, specialist physicians in Ontario went on strike, just as their Quebec counterparts had done for similar reasons in 1970.

While the Canada Health Act may have enshrined a particular notion of national sentiment about health care, it did little to save the Liberal government from resounding defeat to the Progressive Conservatives in the 1984 election. So powerful was its message, however, that no federal government of any political stripe has since challenged or changed its provisions. Still, as significant cuts to federal transfers persisted through the 1990s, concerns were raised about the extent to which the CHA could remain an effective rallying point for publicly funded health care in Canada since its legal purview is limited. More recently, concern has emerged around the "grey areas" of jurisdiction between the Canada Health Act and emerging trends in health care organization and financing across the provinces (Boychuk 2012).

The rest of this chapter approaches the delivery of health care in Canada by describing this delivery through the prism of the Canada Health Act. The chapter also considers how the CHA's principles are reflected in provincial and territorial health systems, explaining how the different components of these systems work and identifying more recent challenges and changes.

The Organization of Health Care in Canada

One way of approaching the organization of health care in Canada is to consider insured health care services as being under the authority of 10 provincial and three territorial systems. Each of these has its own distinct legislation pertaining to hospitals and medical care. Although they are now responsible for the lion's share of health-related spending, all of these governments also avail themselves of federal government transfers tied to certain criteria under the terms of the Canada Health Act. In fact, what these systems have in common is their adherence to the five broad principles underscored in the CHA: public administration, comprehensive coverage of services, universal eligibility, portability across the country, and a guarantee of equal access.

In some cases, these principles are explicitly mentioned in provincial legislation. For example, British Columbia's Medicare Protection Act lays out the five CHA principles one by one, while adding a clause about sustainability. In Ontario, the Commitment to the Future of Medicare Act, passed in 2004, provides powerful endorsement of these principles as well. Other pieces of provincial legislation, for example in Manitoba and Saskatchewan, have less explicit references to the Canada Health Act; the Quebec *Loi sur les services de santé et les services sociaux* has none.

Public administration

As we saw in the previous chapter, each provincial government is the "single payer" through which money flows into their publicly insured health care system. In order for this process to work, provinces must put into place administrative systems that are publicly accountable. Unlike many other public systems in the industrialized world, health care in the Canadian provinces works through an arrangement that allows for public payment, but the services are rendered by entities—hospitals, health care establishments, physicians—not necessarily owned or employed by the state.

For example, the vast majority of hospitals in Canada are considered public, in the sense that their operating revenues come from the single tap of provincial or territorial health departments, usually funnelled through regional agencies or health authorities. Most hospitals across Canada rely on "global budgets" for their operating costs, a system whereby hospitals are accorded yearly funding to cover all of the services they provide. These budgets are typically allocated on the basis of past spending, current needs, and future forecasts, not, as some critics have noted, on performance, quality, or patient satisfaction.

While hospitals are expected to use only public funds for their operating costs (without running deficits), they are not necessarily owned or operated by governments; in fact, hospital ownership can vary—they may be community-based, have a religious vocation or past, be owned by municipal governments, or be part of a university health centre—but they all share a not-for-profit structure. The very few private hospitals that exist in Canada are limited specialized surgery clinics—such as Shouldice Hospital for hernia repair in Toronto—that may provide for-profit services.

Hospitals, then, are governed by their own boards or corporations, although continuous accreditation practices are necessary in order for them to continue to receive funding and to be able to function on behalf of their patients. Still, it means that what happens inside a hospital, such as the organization of services, staff, and providers, is the responsibility of that institution. Sometimes this gives way to certain tensions about responsibilities, such as the recent concerns about the administration of oncological treatments through hospital pharmacies in Ontario.

Physicians in Canada have gone to great lengths to retain their independent status as health care professionals (rather than being considered employees of the state, as are British doctors, for example). Nonetheless, the vast majority of Canadian physicians, whether family physicians or specialists, are part of the publicly funded provincial health care systems, and dependent on provincial governments for virtually all of their income. Typically, a practicing physician in Canada will have been educated and trained through a provincially funded university medical school and its hospital centre. With a licence to practice, the physician is eligible for a billing number, which is used to claim reimbursement from the provincial government or its authorized agency for any medical services rendered to residents registered in the public health services plan. Usually, this is on a fee-for-service basis, with fees set via negotiation between the provincial medical associations and provincial governments, although in Quebec this is done with "federations" that have a quasi-union status in such negotiations. Although physicians are not state employees, their activities are subject to regulation, and for the most part they are required to work exclusively for public payment unless they decide to opt out entirely (relatively few do so). Some exceptions occur; for example, in Manitoba and Alberta, physicians can provide cataract surgery in both public and private facilities.

While physicians negotiate fees through their associations or federations, their regulation as professionals is in the hands of the provincial medical regulatory body that accords their practice licence. In Canada, each province has a College of Physicians and Surgeons (known as the Collège des médecins in Quebec) that acts as a self-regulatory body under provincial law. In addition to licensing and monitoring, such laws empower the colleges to investigate and discipline doctors facing public or professional complaints.

Comprehensive coverage of services

For all of the modern, sophisticated health care services available in Canadian hospitals and by Canadian physicians, the comprehensive benefits covered by provincial health plans tend to be defined in the traditional sense of health care as furnished by physicians and focused on hospital settings. This is reinforced by the Canada Health Act, which stipulates that all "medically necessary" services should be covered by provincial plans. In practice, this means that all in-patient services are covered, including diagnostic procedures, nursing and medical care, any drugs and physiotherapy used in the hospital, all supplies and equipment, too. In addition, all physician outpatient care is covered, offering Canadians a wide array of services, from preventive and primary care to the most sophisticated cutting-edge technology.

And yet, the practice of medicine has changed a great deal over the years, with day surgery, drug therapies, and chronic disease management taking a greater role in treatment and care. Some of these changes have strained the traditional structures of fee-for-service practice by individual physicians, as provinces try to find new remuneration arrangements that can better reflect more integrated and team-based efforts, from primary to tertiary care situations. For example, it would make more sense—in efficiency and financial terms, but also in terms of quality of life—for a vulnerable elderly population to be cared for through a mix of home care, home doctor visits, and regular monitoring through nurse-based telehealth or the intervention of other health care professionals. But publicly funded services tend to be delivered through hospitals or inside doctors' offices. Thus, most vulnerable elderly do not have a coordinated care system they can rely on; instead, they are dependent on office visits, hospital and emergency room care, a family caregiver (for those who have access), or an assisted living situation (for those who can afford it).

Changing medical practices have also meant that the kinds of elements that more and more people rely on for their health care—outpatient drug therapies, home care, long-term care, and the like—may be supplied at an additional cost borne in whole or in part by the individual. Take the example of prescription drug costs. In most provinces, public coverage varies, usually based on criteria such as age or income. Quebec has in place a universal pharmacare program, designed to ensure that every Quebecer has access to some form of insurance coverage for outpatient drugs. In British Columbia, families may register with an income-based pharmacare plan. Ontario has several pharmacare plans in place; these are targeted to the elderly, those with lower incomes, and specific disease groups. For some observers, the absence of a national pharmacare program is a crucial gap in health care for Canadians, leading to a patchwork effect created by provincial coverage, given the increasing importance of drug-related outpatient treatment and the need for better regulation of the growing costs of drugs overall (Daw and Morgan 2012).

Another example can be found in considering conditions that are related to both health and social services. Services for individuals with mental health needs vary greatly from one province to another, as do strategies for diagnosis and treatment. Take autism, for example. Provincial governments have been at a loss in how to deal with the rapidly growing number of cases, since it is hard to ascertain whether this disorder falls under the purview of health, social services, or education, for that matter. And the upshot is that a child with autism, unlike a child with a clear physiological condition, will have access to very different services depending on the province of residence. In British Columbia, a parent-led court challenge attempted to compel the provincial government to cover a controversial and expensive behavioural treatment for autism as a "medically necessary service" (Manfredi and Maioni 2005). Eventually overturned by the Supreme Court, the case raised questions about the scope of government coverage and the locus of decision-making about insured services.

Variation across the provinces can also have important consequences in public health and prevention since, as the adage suggests, "disease knows no borders." This became acutely evident in the aftermath of the severe acute respiratory syndrome (SARS) crisis in Canada. As SARS spread through Toronto-area hospitals in the spring and summer of 2003, attempts to track and contain the epidemic faltered because of the lack of intergovernmental coordination between Ontario and the federal government, and between the provinces themselves. The task force set up to investigate the matter concluded that "Canada's ability to contain an outbreak is only as strong as the weakest jurisdiction in the chain of P/T [provincial-territorial] public health systems" (Naylor and David 2003, 12). The Public Health Agency of Canada was put into place by the federal government in 2004, and part of its mandate was to ensure federal leadership in this area.

Universal eligibility

Most industrialized countries offer a way of ensuring that everyone is eligible for health care services. This is usually done on a "universal" basis, in which the criterion is citizenship or some other form of residency status. In Canada, proof of legal residency in a province or territory is the criterion for eligibility in a public health insurance plan, regardless of age, income, or any other categorical condition. With these conditions in place, no one should fall through the cracks, and 100 percent of Canadians are eligible.

However, there are a number of different population groups whose coverage is mandated through criteria other than provincial residency. These include Aboriginal peoples, military and veterans, federal inmates, and refugees, who are considered the responsibility of the federal government.

This constitutional complexity has often meant that people do fall through the cracks. Historically, the federal government was considered to be responsible for providing care to Aboriginal groups, but as public insurance came into play, physician and hospital services began to be delivered by provinces and territorial governments with the federal government covering the cost. Since the 1980s, there has been a move toward more autonomy for Aboriginal peoples in organizing and staffing community health programs. Today, the federal government's direct role is limited to public health and preventive services for First Nations peoples living on reserves and for Inuit peoples on their traditional territories. In addition, Health Canada also provides supplemental coverage for non–publicly insured services. These benefits, however, do not extend to peoples living off reserve, or to Métis groups. Still, there are persistent gaps in the health outcomes of indigenous peoples, and part of this stems from the difficulty of coordinating care in a policy environment that involves federal and provincial governments, band councils, and remote communities, as well as the need for cultural sensitivity in the development and provision of care.

More recently, there has been a change in coverage for refugees under the Interim Federal Health Program through the categorization of claimants in Canada according to their country of origin. Thus, since 2012, the federal government covers the cost of care only for "government-assisted" refugees; for claimants from countries considered to be "safe," this coverage extends only to urgent care and eliminates supplementary services, such as prescription drugs, unless their condition poses a public health risk. The available evidence suggests that this has increased costs for provinces and territories: some provinces, such as Quebec and Ontario, are extending coverage to these refugees, while other provinces are seeing the impact in emergency rooms and other health care establishments (Barnes 2013).

Portability

The implicit "system" effect that binds together provincial and territorial health plans can be found in the notion of "portability." Simply put, it means that any Canadian, no matter where they find themselves in the country, should be able to access hospital and medical care if needed. So, the Ontario traveller on a ski vacation in British Columbia is covered, as is the Manitoban student who attends university in Nova Scotia. While out-of-province hospital admission are typically examples of urgent care, portability has also come to encompass patient need to access services that may not be available in more remote communities, as is the case in the territories, or patient choice for Canadians living near provincial borders, particularly in the case of childbirth (CIHI 2010).

The problem is that while the notion of portability is federal, its operationalization is tied to interprovincial agreements that are not in the purview of the federal government. In other words, the portability principle depends on voluntary agreements between provinces.

Portability of hospital benefits is thus guaranteed through bilateral reciprocity agreements between the provinces that allow for direct coverage without point-of-service payment required. This also simplifies administrative details for all parties involved. But in the case of outpatient care, things get a bit more complicated. Although provincial health systems do resemble one another in terms of insured services, they are never an exact match, which raises the question of what happens when a patient seeks out-of-province care or consultation that may not be covered by their home provincial plan.

The other, more frequent, complaint is that out-of-province patients may be required to pay for outpatient services up front, and then seek reimbursement from their home health system. Awkward and unwieldy as this may seem for most Canadians, it also leaves Quebecers travelling outside the province in the unenviable situation of being reimbursed only at Quebec rates—typically lower than elsewhere—and having to make up the difference in some way.

Accessibility

In the first years after the establishment of hospital and medical insurance plans, provinces, with the exception of Quebec, tended to allow for certain types of payment to be added on to publicly insured health care services. For example, Ontario and British Columbia allowed physicians (mainly specialists) to extra bill their patients, charging an additional amount over and above the fee schedule. Manitoba and Alberta allowed facility fees to be added on when patients accessed their care in certain health care establishments.

Critics of these fees argued that they imposed financial barriers on access to care, and created an unfair situation in which certain patients could access certain health care providers if they were willing and able to pay more for these services. Thus, when the Canada Health Act was passed in 1984, a new criteria was established in direct response: that each resident have equal access to insured services so that need, not financial ability, remained the principle for distributing resources in the health care sector.

This has been perhaps the most politically charged area of recent health reform debates, because it is a condition that imposes strict financial rules that preclude the development of alternative revenue streams for publicly insured services, for both governments and physicians. Indeed, Quebec had explicitly banned extra billing when it introduced medical care insurance in 1970. As a consequence, specialist physicians broke ranks with the rest of the medical community and went on strike. The strike was unsuccessful, but the province suffered the exodus of a certain number of physicians in the aftermath. When Ontario passed new legislation in 1987 to confirm to the Canada Health Act, another specialist strike was launched.

Accessibility has also been the feature of the Canada Health Act that has received the most attention from the federal government. In the 1990s, the federal government deployed the CHA against British Columbia for allowing extra billing to persist, and against Alberta for allowing clinics to charge facility fees. These actions may have served as a deterrent in the Quebec Liberal government's proposals for emergency room user fees in 1990; however, by 2011 Quebec Liberals were once again considering the possibility of user fees, and criticizing the confines of the Canada Health Act (Maioni 2012).

In practice, equal access means that all insured services are to be delivered on the basis of "first dollar" coverage, without even the smallest of co-payments or fees, so that literally no money changes hands at the point of service with the health care systems. Supplementary private insurance may not cover these publicly funded services, even though, as we have seen, there are several services that remain outside of the public "basket." As the demand for outpatient prescription drugs increases, as does the demand for certain forms of non-urgent care, questions have arisen about what exactly should be included in that public basket of services (Tuohy, Flood, and Stabile 2004).

The Health Care Workforce

Health and health care have a significant impact in the Canadian economy, and constitute an important part of the service sector. In fact, one out of 10 Canadians works in health and social services.

Doctors make up a significant part of that number, and the lion's share of the cost. There are approximately 70,000 physicians in Canada, which translates into about 200 per 100,000 Canadians. This ratio is slightly lower than the Organisation for Economic Co-operation and Development average, although growth in the supply of physicians has recently bounced back from a long decline. Medical school enrollments, which were frozen across the provinces in the 1990s, are now on an upswing as well. How many physicians is enough? It depends, although the evidence suggests it is not just about the numbers, but more importantly about what kind of medicine they practice, the numbers of hours worked, and their geographical distribution.

The other factor in physician care has to do with remuneration. We tend to pay our health care professionals based on the number and type of services they provide, rather than the quality of care or its impact on health outcomes. The vast majority of Canadian doctors still practice on a fee-for-service basis, which gives them considerable autonomy as "private contractors" and allows them a measure of autonomy over their incomes. But fee-for-service payment has its caveats, most importantly the fact that it has the potential for inflation of services and costs, and does little to encourage teamwork.

The upshot is that Canadian physicians are likely to be better remunerated that most of their counterparts in other industrialized countries, with the singular exception of the United States. Because physicians negotiate with provincial agencies, their fees vary across the provinces. Physicians tend to be better remunerated in stronger economic settings such as Alberta and Saskatchewan, and in areas of strong demand such as Ontario, and have historically been less highly paid in Quebec. That being said, the real discrepancies in remuneration have more to do with the differences between family medicine and specialties: in 2010, the average income of a family medicine doctor was in the $240,000 range whereas the specialist was earning an average of $340,000 (CIHI 2013).

Physicians remain among the most mobile of professional groups in Canada, which has meant considerable interprovincial mobility through the years to provinces with booming economies, as well as a preference to practice in urban rather than rural areas. This has led to different strategies to encourage more family physicians to settle in less-serviced rural areas: for example, the establishment of a rural medical school in northern Ontario, and the partial federal loan forgiveness for family doctors in rural settings. Provinces have also tried to deal with this by providing incentives—and disincentives. For example, Quebec has a differential fee schedule in place for new doctors: those who opt to work in rural or remote areas can see their fees increased, while those who remain in "over-serviced" areas may see those fees decreased for the first three to five years of practice.

One trend that has been interrupted is the so-called brain drain of Canadian-trained physicians to the United States; these days, increases in physician salaries have contributed to stem that tide (Hurley and Grant, 2013). In fact, the more pressing problem has to do with foreign medical graduates and whether or not licensing them could alleviate the shortage of physicians to which some critics allude. There is little consensus on this issue for several reasons that have to do with the careful oversight of pan-Canadian and provincial colleges of physicians, the educational interests of Canadian medical schools, the challenges of meshing different training and practice cultures, and the concerns of medical inflation on the part of provincial governments.

Nurses, meanwhile, make up 40 percent of the health care workforce in Canada (CIHI 2013). After important funding cuts led to a decrease in the 1990s, their numbers have been rising steadily in the past few years, especially the numbers of new graduates. There is now a greater potential for foreign-trained nurses to find employment in Canada, and many do choose to follow their career path here, making up about 8 percent of the nursing population. The other trend is the increase in the number of nurse practitioners—much more widely seen in other health care settings, such as the US,—who are able to order diagnostic tests and prescribe drugs.

Challenges and change in health care

The hallmark of "rational" organization of health care systems is rooted in the notion of the differentiation of care into primary, secondary, and tertiary levels according to the volume of demand and acuteness of condition.

It makes sense, since good primary care can be an important part of prevention and health promotion, as well as managing chronic disease and identifying the need for further care. The National Health Service in Britain, for instance, is often cited as an example of such a regimented structure, allowing for a regionalized model of delivery and stepwise patient flow through levels of care (from general practitioner to specialist and hospital).

While provincial and territorial health systems aspire to this type of rationality, it has been difficult to achieve fully integrated health care systems. Some of this is due to unique geographical and demographic factors: remote areas, rural versus urban access, and the like. But some of the barriers have been structural: fee-for-service medicine is seen as problematic for efficient primary care delivery, for maximizing the distribution of physician specialties, and for encouraging more team-based medical models.

Many important reforms in this regard have to do with regionalization of organization and accountability, renewed efforts at primary care reform, and the issue of waiting lists.

Through the 1990s, most of the provinces attempted to decentralize decision-making through the creation of regional health boards (some elected, others appointed, still others a mix of the two). The idea was to allow for more citizen engagement and local input in the allocation of health care resources. There was also the hope of encouraging population-based funding delivery and allocation efficiencies, and defusing tensions about health care budgeting. Some provinces were more successful than others in realizing these goals, and in many provinces, the initial regionalization efforts were later streamlined to bring more coherence to the process.

Primary care reform was spurred by the realization that, although provincial health systems were in theory based on a stepwise access-to-care model, in reality access to services had become dispersed and problematic, with patients seeking care in emergency rooms, walk-in clinics, or with specialists, instead of finding a medical home with a primary caregiver.

The notion of a medical home is anchored in the ideal of a logical entry point into the health care system through the frontline services of primary care. Not only can the majority of health care queries be best addressed through primary care, this approach can also lead to the better management of health needs across the life spectrum. Health systems based on strong primary care models usually have more cost-effective outcomes, healthy populations, and better ways of dealing with the social determinants of health (such as income, housing, and education) in a wider social strategy (Starfield and Shi 2004).

One of the most powerful messages of the 2002 Romanow Report was the recommendation to strengthen primary care across the Canadian provinces. And, indeed, the federal government's subsequent reinvestment in health care spending emphasized the need for primary care reform. Since then, most provinces have moved toward primary care reform strategies, especially Ontario and Quebec (Gutkin 2010).

However, since this is a piecemeal and province-by-province process, the results have not been particularly rapid or sweeping. Family medical groups need physicians and multidisciplinary teams, in short supply in most provinces. The financial incentives for professionals have turned out to be a hefty burden, without (as of yet) a corresponding transformation in the delivery of care.

Even in Quebec, which had long served as a model of integrated health and social service delivery, there remained considerable gaps in the implementation of this principle, and access to primary care physicians had become a problem in urban areas. The formation of family medicine groups, which roster patients, was a response to this, as was the establishment of new networks of care that could bridge more effectively between community services and hospital settings. In Ontario, meanwhile, a long process of primary care reform led to the large-scale expansion of group practice through Family Health Groups and a new capitation payment model for those enrolled in Family Health Organizations (where primary care physicians would be paid for the "global services" provided to a number of patients), along with substantial increases in remuneration for primary care physicians.

Much of the emphasis on regionalization and on primary care reform was intended to inject more efficiency into health care systems in an attempt to assure more appropriate and timely access to care.

Waiting lists for elective surgery, wait times for specialist referrals and diagnostic procedures, and overcrowding of emergency rooms became major political fodder in the late 1990s and early 2000s, symptoms of the larger organizational and funding issues racking provincial health systems. Increased funding from the federal government and an overall improved economic picture in most of the provinces has alleviated some of this, but the political repercussions remain important.

The substantial public furor over wait times was reflected in federal election campaigns in the mid-2000s, as health reform topped voter concerns and electoral saliency. The spectacle of emergency rooms crowded by stretchers and hours of waiting made regular media headlines across the provinces.

In fact, the whole notion of access to care has now widened to include the issue of timeliness. Even though, as many analysts have pointed out (see Aaron and Swartz 1990), allocating relatively high-demand but also very expensive resources such as health care requires decisions that inevitably lead to some form of rationing, public opinion expresses dissatisfaction with waiting for consultations, diagnostics, and elective surgeries. The 2002 Senate report on the federal role in health care explicitly identified wait times as a barrier in access to care, and recommended the enactment of a "health care guarantee" for timely treatment.

And waiting times for elective surgery were at the heart of a 2005 Supreme Court decision, *Chaoulli v. Quebec*, which ruled that Quebec could not ban private insurance for core medical services if that meant undue waiting times in access to care in the public system; the scathing criticism by the Chief Justice Beverley McLachlin was that "access to a waiting list is not access to health care." It was a divided decision, but one that reflected not only the importance of wait times as a matter of public debate but also the growing impact of the courts in health policy conflicts.

Conclusion

Perhaps the greatest paradox of health care in Canada is that, despite myths about a single system of care in a very decentralized landscape, we have, after all, ended up with a relatively coherent mosaic instead of a crazy quilt of different programs across the provinces and territories.

Still, even with widespread eligibility, extensive coverage, and relatively equal access to care, it is a mosaic that is facing considerable pressure to adapt and reform. Some of this pressure stems from enduring challenges in the way care is delivered, such as in remote and rural populations, the specific needs of indigenous peoples, and the quest for a medical home through primary care reform. Other pressures stem from new challenges in the provision of care and the growth of non-insured services, the need to better manage chronic care, the growing expectations and dissatisfaction in public opinion, and the ever-looming need to adapt delivery and organization to meet the needs of an aging society.

While these challenges may be felt across Canada, the fact remains that they will be addressed at the level of provincial policy-making. We may see attempts at interprovincial coordination, and hopefully better strategies for cross-provincial learning, but in the absence of a framework for federal leadership in this policy area, the onus is on provincial governments to face the challenges of health care reform in the 21st century.

Chapter 3

The Facts about Health Care Spending

Of all the conundrums in health care, perhaps the most puzzling has to do with financing. How much, in effect, is enough or too much? What financing principles should guide the distribution of care? And who should be paying the costs?

Money is a difficult issue to address, especially when it comes to health care. Part of the problem is that such a discussion can quickly get out of control—money and taxes are touchy subjects at the best of times, and even more so when we are dealing with the billions of dollars it costs to deliver health care services to Canadians. But the other part of the problem is that it is hard to grasp the real meaning of the cost of health care when we talk about the huge sums of money involved in government spending, public budgets, and the like.

To bring these topics into a more meaningful focus, this chapter begins with a story about the pocketbook issues of money and health. And, in this case, it is my own story. Like most women, my first extended contact with the health care system centred on a first pregnancy. What should have been a relatively simple primigravida quickly became a more serious medical issue. The ensuing bed rest, Caesarean section operation, and weeks of neonatal intensive care were carried out in a hospital setting with sophisticated technology and unfailing professional excellence. At the end of this months-long odyssey, I was handed a bill for $18, the cost of a phone in my hospital room.

This is the point in the story where most American observers would gasp, since the "real" cost of all that care was undoubtedly in the six figures. So, the first lesson of health care spending in Canada is relatively straightforward: through provincial health plans, the costs of specific care are factored into a larger redistribution across the health care system, controlled by hospital budgets and negotiated professional fees. In insurance terms, since risk is spread across a large and varied population, what could have been a ruinous financial situation for an individual taxpayer family was absorbed across the system.

Fast forward a few years to another situation in which one of my children is diagnosed with severe autism. Here, at the fringes of the health care system—that is, outside of a health care establishment and away from physician hands—the financial story is very different. The diagnosis of this medical condition came from a hospital, but most of the significant costs of care since then (prescription drugs, psychology, occupational therapy, speech therapy, etc.) have been borne in other ways, ways that rely on supplemental insurance and out-of-pocket spending. Which leads to a second lesson about health spending in Canada: not everything medically diagnosed is covered by the public system, and the private-spending portion can be a heavy financial burden.

Let's face it: there is nothing free about health care, in Canada as elsewhere. Canadians pay a substantial price for services they value and use. In so doing, they contribute to insuring themselves against the cost of sickness, relaying resources from the healthy to the sick, and, at the same time, effecting a broader redistribution across income groups. Because the lion's share of money flows through the public purse, governments and their agencies have a great deal of leverage over the rules of the financing game, and some measure of cost control as well. Still, the burden on the public sector is substantial and growing. The rest of this chapter examines the mix of health care financing modes in Canada and the mechanics of the single-payer system in a federal polity.

Hey, Big Spender?

There are three main questions we can address with regard to health care spending in Canada. First, how much is being spent? Second, what is the money being spent on? And finally, who exactly is paying?

In comparative terms, Canada is a "big spender" in health care, part of the top-tier group of industrialized countries that now spend just over 10 percent of their GDP (gross domestic product) on health care. Germany and France, for example, spend about 11 percent of GDP on health care, while the US spends considerably more, almost 17 percent. (All data in this chapter is from the Canadian Institute for Health Information, unless otherwise specified.)

Health care now accounts for somewhere between 11 percent and 12 percent of the total of all goods and services in Canada. What this means is that over $200 billion is being spent on health and health care in Canada. In per capita terms, in 2012 this translated into $6,000 per person, although it is worth noting that this amount varies across the provinces. At the lowest end, it is $5,500 in Quebec, and it reaches a high of $7,000 in Newfoundland. Costs in the territories are even higher. Still, this is within the range of many industrialized countries, and considerably less than the US. When Canadian amounts are translated into comparable figures (by adjusting for purchasing power parity), per capita spending is estimated at $4,500 in Canada. Compare this to nearly $8,000 in the US, where nearly $3 trillion is spent on health care per year.

And health costs are rising in Canada. This is largely the result of increased demand for and volume of services provided, plus advances in medicine that include pricier technologies and pharmaceutical costs. To understand the drivers of health care costs, we can compare our current spending with that of the past. In 1975, health care accounted for 7 percent of GDP. As we saw above, that figure has since risen to somewhere around 12 percent.

There are several ways to better understand this significant growth. First, it is worth noting that there have been variations within that time. The Canadian Institute for Health Information, for example, breaks down three distinct periods since 1975: significant growth in spending from 1976 to 1991, as governments expanded health care systems; retrench-ment from 1992 to 1996, which coincided with significant cuts in fed-eral transfers to the provinces; and reinvestment from 1997 to 2008, as governments focused on meeting popular expectations, and the federal-provincial 10-year plan kicked in (CIHI 2011).

More recently, health care costs have outpaced inflation, increasing overall at about 3.4 percent from 2000 to 2010, with a slowing of growth after the 2008 recession. Much of that can be attributed to higher spending in the public sector, during the period of reinvestment by provinces and the federal government. But this is linked to the increase in overall prices in the health sector—the cost drivers—to pay for hospitals and their functioning, to pay for physician fees, and to pay for in-patient and outpatient diagnos-tic testing and prescription drugs.

At the time that publicly funded hospital and medical insurance came into effect in the provinces, the average Canadian would have interacted with the health care system in the context of a life event (such as child-birth), an accident, or an illness. Far fewer people than today would have been treated for chronic conditions, complicated and rare diseases and complex disabilities, or would have sought out elective surgeries. And hos-pitals and physicians were much more limited in the kinds of care, medica-tion, diagnostic testing, and technology available to them. This is no longer the case. Today, as the frontiers of medical research grow ever wider, as the expectations of patients and their families continue to escalate, and as the costs of technology increase steadily, health care has become a very big business, indeed.

Perhaps understanding the long-term trends in health care spending involves more than looking at a spreadsheet of spending over time. The other change we can chart is what this money has been spent on. In earlier days, the lion's share of health care expenditures went to pay for hospitals and physicians. As the delivery of care has changed over time, so too has the way money is spent in the health care system. Today, hospitals account for about 30 percent of health expenditures, while other health care establishments (such as long-term care facilities) make up 10 percent of the total. Physician fees and payment are 14 percent, while other health care professionals account for another 10 percent. And drug costs have increased to almost 16 percent, a marked increase from just a few decades ago.

But in order to really understand the financing of health care in Canada, it is also important to figure out who is actually paying. This brings us to the enduring conflict in the debate over health care in Canada about public versus private spending. The moniker of a single-payer system in Canada may conjure up tight regulation and extensive public control, but the reality is somewhat different. First of all, the "single payer" isn't so single, after all: the term refers to provincial governments, not a sole government nor the federal government. The public payments that flow through these single taps account for 70 percent of the total amount of spending in the health care sector, even though these payments are made to ostensibly private actors, such as physicians, who are not employees of the state. In other words, it is the source of funds that is public, not necessarily the services that are being paid for.

In addition, it is important to remember that 30 percent of total health spending in Canada—a relatively high proportion when compared to most comparator countries—is actually spent outside the public system. This is due to the fact that the "basket" of insured services covered by provincial health care plans includes medically necessary care, generally defined as care provided in a hospital or health care establishment, and in the hands of a licensed professional physician. But the basket does not necessarily include services rendered outside of this definition (think physiotherapy, for example) or delivered outside of an establishment (such as some diagnostic testing). Also not included is self-administered care (such as outpatient pharmaceuticals) or the care provided by certain professionals (such as dental care).

While costs are increasing overall in the health care system, there are important pressures in these services, in particular the price of drug therapies and diagnostic testing. And these non-insured services also represent the part of the health care system where access is different for Canadians based on their supplementary insurance coverage or ability to pay out of pocket for things that are not covered by the public plan, such as outpatient prescription drugs in some provinces, and dental care in most provinces.

Follow the Money

How does money flow through the health care system? The image of a single payer can help illustrate this process. Essentially, the provincial government collects revenue—through its own sources, federal government transfers, equalization payments, and, in some provinces (Ontario, British Columbia, and Quebec) via direct premiums on residents. This revenue is then distributed—with the provincial government acting as the single payer (as opposed to multiple insurance payers, as is the case in the United States, for example)—for public health initiatives and health care services.

Then we can consider how funding flows from provincial treasuries into health care consumption by individual users. Provincial funding flows through two main streams. The first of these is to pay for hospitals and health care establishments. Hospitals in Canada are defined as not-for-profit institutions, which means that they are not in the business of making profits for shareholders. As such, they provide services through the funds allocated to them, attempting to walk that fine line between surplus and deficit. These funds generally take the form of annual "global budgets" that are allocated to hospitals and health care establishments, usually through regional health authorities on the basis of a mix of retrospective and prospective accounting. But this kind of funding does not really provide much in the way of incentives for hospitals to organize themselves more efficiently or even to provide quality care. Some provinces, in particular Ontario, have experimented with activity-based funding, which is supposed to allocate money based on the kinds of patients and volume of services provided by each hospital. Thus, the emphasis is on the care actually provided based on patient diagnosis, not general expenditures.

The second main stream of public funding goes to pay the doctors. Against all odds (and trends in other countries), the reimbursement of physicians in Canada has remained entrenched in the fee-for-service model, where fees are paid to professionals through fee schedules negotiated with physician associations or their representatives. Historically speaking, this is considered the "compromise" that allowed publicly funded medical insurance to see the light of day across the provinces: doctors agreed to be part of the system as long as they could retain professional and financial autonomy through their billing practices. The critiques of fee-for-service are legion: by offering a payment for every single medical act, fee-for-service is said to create incentives for volume, rather than quality of care; it creates disincentives for collaborative care; and it may even lead to unnecessary or inappropriate care.

Many other kinds of reimbursement schemes are being touted to remedy the fee-for-service gridlock. These include capitation, pay-for-performance (which would reward appropriate and cost-effective care), or some form of mixed payment that would allow physicians to bundle the costs of caring for the specific needs of a patient (Léger 2011). We see evidence of these approaches in many provinces, especially in primary care settings: blended payments through family health or medicine groups in Ontario and Quebec; capitation experiments in Alberta; and the possibility of a fixed-salary model for community-based family doctors in most provinces.

Whatever the arrangement, the cost implications are considerable, which is why negotiations between provinces and physicians often become a battle of wills and, increasingly, a battle for public opinion. Provincial governments have tended to see physicians as a major part of the medical inflation problem; physicians, on the other hand, demand to be reimbursed as highly qualified professionals, in demand on a global scale. And, as Picard (2013) has noted, physicians (like hospitals) generate over $30 billion in tax revenues for governments. Today, physicians are among the highest-paid income group in Canada. Still, since they are not allowed to accept any payment other than public reimbursement unless they decide to opt out entirely, this means that their income is generated almost exclusively from the public coffers.

Where does this money come from? We noted above that individuals themselves pay for health care in a number of different ways. They pay federal taxes and provincial taxes, which find their way into provincial general revenues; they also pay through consumption taxes, such as sales taxes. Still, there is a lot more money sloshing around in the health care system than the amounts devoted to hospitals and physicians through public treasuries. Individual Canadians may also be paying a monthly premium for supplementary insurance against the items that are not covered by their provincial plan: prescription drugs, optometrist fees and eyeglasses, physiotherapy, private nursing care, and the like. In so doing, they are likely also paying out-of-pocket for co-payments and other kinds of fees associated with these expenses. In some provinces, certain types of diagnostic testing may be available more rapidly if patients have supplementary insurance or are willing to pay directly for these services.

And who gets what, overall? The so-called demographic tsunami is often cited as a cost driver. As Canada's population ages, the effects on the health care system will be substantial. This is true in practically all of its aspects—from the cost of drugs to the availability of services, and from the aging of the health care workforce to the impact on family care providers. In effect, Canadians aged 65 and older make up over 40 percent of provincial spending on health care; infants are also a relatively high-expenditure group, given the volume of births relative to other in-hospital procedures, and also due to the high costs of treating infant-related intensive care situations.

Still, much of the scientific evidence provides a cautionary tale about falling into the correlation traps that saddle an aging population with an increased spending on health care. An aging population undoubtedly puts pressures on the health care system, but the impact of aging cannot be isolated as a cost driver per se. First, the impact of aging on costs varies across regions and depends on the overall demographic structure of the population. Second, and more pertinent still, the chronic diseases associated with aging are the main drivers of costs. As Canadians live longer today than in the past, the challenge really becomes how to reform the provision of appropriate (and more cost-effective) care for this population through a better organization of hospital and long-term care, home and community care, and palliative care. It also means coming to terms with the fact that in most provinces, much of this care falls outside the publicly insured system, leaving individual Canadians and their families even more vulnerable.

Pressures on Provincial Treasuries

From the discussion above, it's obvious that health care presents real money challenges. These challenges are becoming more pronounced as our lifespans increase, new drugs and other medical technologies become available, and economic growth is increasingly fragile.

These challenges are becoming more and more intense for public treasuries across Canada. Public spending in health care amounts to billions of dollars and requires enormous sums of money for provincial governments.

The nature of Canadian federalism complicates matters, since it is provinces that are responsible for health services, even though all of them rely on additional federal monies to meet their obligations. This type of arrangement has considerable benefits. It allows policy diversity across a vast country in which regions do not share the same population demographic, fiscal or physical landscape, or potential for generating revenues. And it allows provinces the ability to use their particular institutional features to shape public policy as they see fit. But there are drawbacks, too. Federalism makes the notion of "pan-Canadian" measures or strategies in health outcomes, quality assessment, even evidence-based policy-making in health care more difficult to develop and assess. It also means that the kinds of policy learning or economies of scale that could result from more intense interaction between health care systems have yet to be realized. Add to this the fact that health care represents a sensitive area for politicians of all partisan stripes—it is fraught with the minefields of public opinion and accountability, and it serves as a lightning rod for federal-provincial conflict—and you have a recipe for considerable controversy and confusion.

Provincial governments are being squeezed in two ways over health care costs. Since provincial governments are responsible for a number of social policy areas, they must rely on general revenues to finance a wide array of programs, including health, social services, and education. It has been estimated that, on average, provinces now spend about 40 percent of their total program spending on health care. Thus, governments have claimed that increased expenditures in health care are crowding out other program spending, jeopardizing their ability to provide social programs and threatening the fiscal stability of provincial treasuries. In more concrete terms, economists talk about the spending pie and the ever-increasing slice, or bite, represented by health care. Other observers find this metaphor misleading, since the pie itself has shrunk over time as governments cut back on the ingredients for revenue-generating, such as taxes.

Whatever the metaphor, the message is the same: health care is pressuring provincial budgets and may in some cases be redirecting spending from other social sectors. In political science terms, it is easy to trace the power dynamics at play: provincial governments are exposed to heavy pressure from powerful interest groups, namely physicians and unions representing public-sector health care workers, while at the same time conscious of patient interests and public opinion.

Beyond this lies the concern about another type of pie: the one that represents the share of the costs of health care between the provinces and the federal government. Provinces have seen their share of the total health care cost burden rise rapidly over the past few decades. As the historical record points out, the federal government initiated cost-sharing programs as a way of inducing the provinces to invest in health care and set up public insurance plans. The original shared-cost programs in hospital and medical care that emerged in the 1950s and 1960s were replaced with block grants in the 1970s; these, in turn, were chipped away through the 1990s, until the fiscal boost of the 2003–04 health accords. Provinces use these transfers and their own revenue sources (which may include equalization payments) in the funding equation. When public health and other health-related spending by the federal government is added into the mix, it becomes difficult to accurately estimate which level of government pays for what share of the health care costs that flow through the public system. Nevertheless, it is clear that the notion of cost-sharing has been phased out over time.

The Paradox of Fiscal Federalism

The tension between provincial and federal governments over health care spending can be attributed to two factors. On the one hand, there is a constitutional paradox. The federal government has, over time, developed a strong fiscal muscle in its capacity to tax and spend. Meanwhile, provinces have seen their jurisdictional reach widen as many of the key responsibilities of the modern state have been interpreted from the rather sketchy wording of Section 92 of the Constitution Act. In light of this paradox—federal fiscal capacity versus provincial jurisdictional responsibility—there has emerged the claim that the federal government needs to be more generous in its fiscal transfers so that provinces can ensure health care services for their residents. On the other hand, there is balance between who pays and who gets to make the rules. Hence, the concept of the "golden rule" in fiscal federalism: the federal government, through its fiscal largesse or "gold," gets to have some political clout in laying down the "rules" of how that money is to be spent by the provinces. For equalization payments, which flow directly into the general revenues of eligible provinces, the point is moot, but for direct federal transfers to provincially administered social programs and health care, the concept of the golden rule persists.

As was pointed out in a previous chapter, many provinces were wary of publicly funded health care, some due to the fears of a fiscal burden, others to the potential of having to play by federal rules. These fears were assuaged to some extent by the federal government's initiative in setting up shared-cost mechanisms within a loose framework for the provinces. But even within the federal government, there were substantial misgivings about the fiscal commitment taken on (painstakingly detailed in Taylor and Paget 1989). The original design of these cost-shared programs in hospital and medical care was fundamentally altered through the introduction of the Established Programs Financing (EPF) Act of 1977 (covering hospital, medical, and postsecondary education payments). What had previously been open-ended spending formulae—that is, provincial governments were essentially reimbursed on a cost-shared basis for their health care expenditures—was replaced with block grants that were essentially decided upon by the federal government, and distributed to the provinces on a per capita population basis. This meant that provinces were now responsible for budgeting and cost containment.

As the fiscal picture worsened through the 1980s, subsequent Progressive Conservative governments restricted the growth in these transfers, and then froze them after 1989. Provincial governments soon found themselves squeezed by the economic effects of recession, reduced transfers, and increasing pressure on social programs. By the mid-1990s, the

federal deficit situation had grown so dire that the new Liberal government decided to entirely rewrite the fiscal transfer map, replacing the EPF
arrangements and the Canada Assistance Plan with a mammoth Canada
Health and Social Transfer. The impact on provincial health systems was
immediate and intense, with negative growth in spending, hospital clos-
ings, and, in some cases, rapid restructuring of delivery as well.

As the economic situation improved, the 1999 federal budget promised the injection of significant monies over five years to provincial health
transfers. In 2000, a health care funding agreement further increased transfers to the provinces, with a guaranteed minimum, but still left provincial leaders concerned about their fiscal capacity to meet increasing health
care costs. In 2003, a new Canada Health Transfer (CHT) was introduced,
along with a Health Reform Fund intended to fund targeted initiatives
(Primary Health Care, Home Care, Catastrophic Drugs, and Diagnostic
and Medical Equipment). These had been highlighted in the 2002 report
of the Commission on the Future of Health Care (the Romanow Report).

After extensive negotiations at a high-profile First Ministers' meeting in
2004, the federal government and the premiers reached an agreement on
multi-year, stable health care funding. Prime Minister Paul Martin, who
as finance minister had been the architect of the 1995 cuts, committed
the federal government to a 10-year plan for increased health care transfers. In all, the federal government estimated this would inject $41 bil-
lion into health care across Canada through immediate cash increases in
2004–05, an annual 6 percent increase as of 2006–14, and a Wait Times
Reduction Transfer. The latter had been highlighted in the Senate Standing
Committee report of 2002, and would be reinforced by the *Chaoulli v.
Quebec* decision in 2005.

These increases allowed the provinces to raise overall spending, but also,
ostensibly, to tackle long-overdue primary care reform and to address the
waiting times problem. Both of these became thorny issues at the implementation stage on the ground in the provinces, and the 10-year anniver-
sary of the 2004 accord will surely bring up the question of accountability
over the monies spent during the past decade.

Meanwhile, the Conservative government in Ottawa has signalled that it
is not interested in getting into another fiscal food fight with the provinces.
Instead of engaging in the high politics of another round of negotiations, it
was left to the finance minister, Jim Flaherty, to make a surprise announce-
ment in December 2011 at a meeting of his provincial counterparts. Then
and there, without fanfare or formal provincial input, the federal government signalled its intention to wind down these former spending commit-
ments: first, by extending the 6 percent escalator through the 2016–17
fiscal year; and then, by returning to a health transfer calculation based on

economic growth as measured by GDP (the original foundation of block funding in 1977). For the Conservative government, then, the ball for cost control will move squarely onto the provinces' side of the court.

The "Golden Rule"

These health accords and injections of federal funding considerably defused intergovernmental tensions. And the pressures of the "golden rule" have been assuaged by the coming to power of a Conservative government (after 2006) much less interested in flexing its political muscle in health care than its Liberal predecessors.

When shared-cost programs came into being, the rules of the game were not spelled out as they are today. The 1957 Hospital Insurance and Diagnostic Services Act included "informal conditions" for federal payment, while the Medical Care Act of 1966 alluded to a "federal-provincial understanding." This included criteria such as allowing for portability across provinces, a reasonably comprehensive range of services offered by provincial plans, a guarantee that every resident of Canada would be covered by a provincial plan, and public accountability for the money spent. Still, many observers—including Emmett Hall, the author of the 1964 Royal Commission report that spurred federal medical insurance—concluded that provincial governments were jeopardizing access to health care services by tolerating extra billing by physicians and user charges imposed by establishments. The passage of the Canada Health Act in 1984 was designed to change that. It's purpose was "to establish criteria and conditions in respect of insured health services and extended health care services provided under provincial law that must be met before a full cash contribution may be made" (CHA 1985, 3). The act identified five precise criteria that provinces would need to meet in order to qualify for that contribution.

The CHA was a short document, economical in words but explosive in its impact. The political impact was immediate, as provinces like Ontario were forced to change their own legislation to conform. And during the 1990s, the federal government deployed the act in a few instances to rein in the provinces, such as British Columbia. Still, the main impact was symbolic. The CHA became associated with a political "space" for the federal government as the protector of a popular social program. It also heightened conflict with Quebec, which chafed at the idea of federal rules imposed in its own area of jurisdiction. In 1991, the Quebec government mused about user fees in hospital emergency rooms; a more recent example was the 2011 Quebec budget, which proposed a *ticket orienteur*: a retroactive fee of $25 per medical visit assessed through income tax filing, and adjusted for income. Although the Quebec Liberal government claimed the proposal was not in violation of the Canada Health Act (since access was not compromised at the point of contact with the delivery of services), the budget did explicitly state that the "Canada Health Act should not impede the search for solutions that will ensure long-term funding for our healthcare system" (Quebec 2010, iv). Highly controversial, the *ticket* was never implemented.

Future Costs and Directions

In the past few years, there has been relative quiet on the fiscal federal front, as health care became less of a tension-filled political lightning rod. Much of this is due to the fact that public opinion and provincial reaction has been favourably influenced by the federal government's largesse. This may change after 2014, as the 10-year accord winds down, and depending on the fiscal situation in Canada and the political stripes of the government in power.

This wary peace, however, has not obscured the real challenges facing provincial governments when it comes to investing in health care reform, nor has it alleviated the pressure for them to either ramp up revenues for health care or move more firmly toward cost-control measures. Some of this can be seen in the recent initiatives of provincial governments to collaborate in planning for the future through the Council of the Federation's working groups in health care innovation and financing.

While spending rather than saving seemed to be the leitmotif of the Canadian health care sector in the 2000s, the 2008 recession served to focus the minds of politicians and the public alike about some of the long-term challenges facing the system. And, recession or not, the actual amount of money spent on health care in Canada has doubled since the mid-1990s—from $100 billion to $200 billion per year, and most of it is taxpayer money.

Beyond the question of how much health care costs is the enduring question of how to pay for it. Despite the caricatural nature of some of the debates around health care costs as a battle between public and private or between single-payer and two-tiered medicine, the reality of the funding issues is much more complex. For some observers, the solution is to move more firmly toward cost control within the public system—more efficient hospital organization, better control of physician costs—and to extend this control to other areas of the health care system, such as a outpatient drug coverage through pharmacare—in other words, to expand the basket of insured health services so as to effect a broader control on total costs.

For these observers, one thing is certain: costs may be contained, but they will continue to rise. The advances of medical science, research, and technology are such that we can barely imagine what transformations are next. But we can imagine that we will want to have access to them in the most affordable way possible. The question is how to allocate these scarce resources for which, in theory, there is no real limit, if we assume that staying healthy or being cured has no price.

For others, the solution means finding alternative revenue sources within the public system, such as user fees or co-payments, or other public-private arrangements that could loosen demand on the public system for certain services. Beyond this, there have been proposals for new, separate kinds of mandatory insurance (for catastrophic costs related to aging, for example) or special investments by governments for innovation funding.

And yet, putting user fees on services is hardly a revolutionary change, nor will the potential revenue generated offset either the administrative costs involved or the risks for price-sensitive patients—usually the most vulnerable, too. Private funding of health care services is no more efficient than public; in fact, all the evidence actually points to the opposite conclusion. Loosening the bonds of payment for physicians and hospitals brings us to similar brick walls unless these alternative revenues are designed to explicitly encourage collaborative arrangements that can lead to better health outcomes. So far, the evidence is far from conclusive in this regard, and the relative scarcity of health human resources means that is unlikely to ever be.

We are now beset with studies on how we can "bend the cost curve," but a more fundamental question is why we are engaged in a debate about who should pay for what in health care. For now, among Canadians, there seems to be a general consensus that the "best" way to allocate care is on the basis of need rather than the ability to pay, which means redistributing risk, care, and costs across a wide population and fiscal base. This consensus was sorely tested when cost-control mechanisms were introduced without well-thought-out rigour or reason in the 1990s, and it will likely be sorely tested again if governments and providers are unable to address the needs for better coordination and reform efforts for Canada's future challenges.

What will those challenges be? This chapter began with a series of medical vignettes, the same sort that are repeated many times over each and every day in the health care system: access to routine procedures, the urgent need for more serious interventions, and the ongoing care of chronic conditions. Similar situations, some of them yours, are to be found across all age groups, all income groups, and all regions of Canada. All of these involve trade-offs in terms of who gets what, when, and how. And they all involve substantial amounts of money.

Indeed, the question that Canadians need to answer is not simply how much governments can "afford" to spend on health care; individuals are doing the spending, after all, whether through taxes to fund publicly insured services or by paying for other types of services themselves. What governments can do is provide the structure to ensure that the most appropriate quality of care and the most cost-effective care is being delivered.

The more complex question is to what extent Canadians are willing to continue to allow governments to set out those markers and regulate the payment and provision of care. Do Canadians want to push for better regulation and coordination of health care services that they already pay for? Will they accept what this may mean for the allocation of scarce resources for the public good?

The answers to these questions depend on many things, not the least of which is personal preference in the context of societal needs. And Canadians are not alone in facing these issues. Across the world, countries are grappling with the challenge of cost containment in the face of increased demand for health care services. The next two chapters outline these comparative stories and how they may inform the debate over health reform in Canada.

Chapter 4

Why No National Health Insurance in the United States?

President Barack Obama's recent engagement on health care legislation in the United States must be seen as part of a continuum of presidential efforts designed to move toward the difficult goal of health reform. It should also be understood as part of a very difficult historical trajectory. From the feisty offence plays of Harry Truman through to Bill Clinton's all-out efforts, the domestic agenda of US politics carries the battle scars of that great, unfinished business: universal health insurance for all Americans.

The absence of a universal, national health insurance program in the United States offers an intriguing policy puzzle—not just for policy scholars but also for Canadian observers of the US more generally (Maioni 1998). Even though, as Jeff Simpson has opined, "the U.S. model offers an unfortunate distraction and a false comparison" (Simpson 2012, 10), the fact remains that the American experience is particularly compelling for a Canadian audience, sharing a cross-border proximity of ideas and images about health care. And the comparison is all the more useful given our shared cultural and economic spheres, not to mention a common history of medical care delivery.

It's true that spiralling health costs, pressures for fiscal reform, and problems of access and quality are concerns for industrialized nations beyond North America, but in no other country has the basic legitimacy of the right to health care (and affordable health insurance) been subject for so long to such fundamental scrutiny or attack as in the United States. Nowhere is this more evident than in the case of health insurance.

The American Experience

The remarkable exceptionalism of the United States in health policy is even more intriguing given that the quest for health insurance stretches back to the early decades of the 20th century, well before Canadian interest in the matter. During the Progressive Era in the mid-1910s, European precedents had convinced many American social reformers and medical professionals that health insurance was "inevitable" (Starr 1982). The first attempts to promote government involvement were led by former president Theodore Roosevelt, who formally endorsed compulsory health insurance as leader of the Bull Moose Progressive Party in 1912. More plausible were the state-level initiatives (particularly strong in California), but as they were based on the German social insurance model, they were denounced as "foreign" infiltration, and did not survive World War I.

The election of Franklin Roosevelt in 1932 and his determination to actively respond to the Great Depression would lay the basis for the Social Security Act (SSA) of 1935 and affirm federal leadership in American social policy. Roosevelt's hand-picked group of economic advisors showed interest in designing health insurance, but the president was keenly aware of its vulnerability alongside the proposals for old age pensions, social assistance, and unemployment insurance (Witte and Perkins 1962). Health insurance was eventually left out of the 1935 bill, due in large part to the opposition of business and the medical profession allied with conservative interests in Congress. Nonetheless, the Social Security Act was groundbreaking legislation: nothing in Canada at the time could compare. Unlike the vacuum that existed in Canada, the provisions of the SSA would have a resounding impact on the future path of health reform in the United States.

Roosevelt returned, belatedly, to health insurance once the Great Depression was over. As World War II wore on, Roosevelt became intrigued by British discussions of postwar reconstruction and the notion of "cradle-to-grave" security (which intimates credited to him, not to Lord Beveridge, see Perkins 1946). Cautious about translating this vision into legislation, it was not until the 1944 presidential campaign in the final months of war that Roosevelt focused on an Economic Bill of Rights, including the right to medical care

When Harry Truman was left to carry on Roosevelt's work, he was determined to maintain existing social programs to highlight the continuity in leadership, and to champion health insurance as a way of carving out his own reform legacy through his Fair Deal. Unlike his predecessor, Truman was prepared to forge ahead despite the controversy surrounding health insurance. The former "straight-ticket" New Deal senator was aware of the opposition, particularly from the medical lobby, but as his contemporaries noted, that did not stop him (Altmeyer 1966). On November 19, 1945, Truman presented an historic message to Congress on health reform, the first president to ever do so, emphasizing the link to Roosevelt's call for "freedom from want." His proposals (including investment in hospital construction, public health, medical training and research, and a plan for "prepayment of medical costs") were endorsed by many groups, including organized labour, and for a time enjoyed substantial public support (Poen 1979). By the end of the decade, however, only the Hospital Survey and Construction Act of 1946 had been passed.

The hostility to health insurance in Congress was palpable, not only among Republicans but also more acutely within Democratic ranks. The conservative coalition that had emerged in opposition to the New Deal grew ever more powerful as southern Democrats flexed their political muscle against the Fair Deal for a variety of reasons, including blocking anything that would affect states' autonomy and race relations (Boychuk 2008). These Dixiecrats, as they were known, targeted Truman and his like-minded reformers in the Congress.

Meanwhile, the formidable Senate leader, Robert Taft, attacked health and social reform as part of his isolationist position; it was also indicative of his fears about socialism and communism. The spectre of "socialized medicine" turned out to be a particularly lurid image in the context of the nascent Cold War. This ideologically charged opposition was aided by the onslaught of an extensive public relations campaign led by the American Medical Association (Starr 1982).

Truman tried no less than three times to press forward health insurance legislation, but as with Bill Clinton, his failure would be a crucial factor in the Republican's regaining of Congress and, eventually, the presidency. It would also be the reason that the Democratic leadership was wary of re-embarking on a doomed path.

The sustained opposition by organized medicine and in Congress forced reformers to refocus their attempts on something more politically feasible. The Social Security Act had set the precedent of "entitlement"—that is, access to certain government programs based on specific criteria of age. Since the elderly were in essence a non-controversial political constituency and a "deserving" clientele, it made sense to focus efforts on the clientele of a widely popular federal program (Marmor 1983).

Moreover, the elderly were becoming a powerful lobby in their own right, and the importance of the "rocking chair" vote was apparent. In the absence of government health insurance initiatives, employer-based bene-fits and private insurance were filling the vacuum, leaving the elderly as the most vulnerable to the effects of ill health and medical costs. The move toward this entitlement approach would become the defining difference between the US and other countries, such as Canada, that instead embraced the notion of universal coverage and eligibility.

From this targeted strategy emerged the proposals that would lead to President John F. Kennedy's appeal for health insurance legislation for the aged in the face of concerted opposition from the medical and insurance professions, even as the polls were showing widespread public support. His efforts went down to defeat in the Senate, and it would take three more years, and a significant shift in the composition of the Congress, for Medicare to finally see the light of day in the US.

Labelled "the foot in the door to socialized medicine" by its opponents, health insurance for the aged would become part of Lyndon Johnson's Great Society program after the breakthrough 1964 election that brought Democratic majorities to the House and Senate. With the concerted bipartisan politicking for which Congress is so famous, a compromise was passed in the form of an amendment to the Social Security Act. It included a social insurance program for hospital insurance for the elderly (Medicare Part A), and a supplementary medical insurance plan (Medicare Part B). At the same time, an existing program that had provided assistance to the very poor elderly was replaced by Medicaid, a federal-state partnership that would allow states to cover the medically indigent—mainly welfare recipients.

It was not without reluctance that US reformers turned away from "universal" health insurance, but at the time, the 1965 breakthroughs were considered a beginning rather than an end (Marmor 1983). As the years wore on, however, this retreat from universality would become the most important distinguishing feature from the Canadian approach. The Social Security Act had set the precedent for age-based cleavages in social benefits, and reinforced the idea of "deserving" groups. In Canada, no such precedent was ever firmly institutionalized. While reform efforts would begin with hospital insurance, and be followed by medical care, the universality principle held firm.

Through Medicare and Medicaid, the US government took on the responsibility to guarantee access to health care for those groups most likely to be shut out of the voluntary and employer-based market for health insurance in the United States. In other words, government was relegated to the role of insuring groups with the highest actuarial risk. Although both insurance interests and the medical lobby were initially hostile to such reforms, they were given important roles in the organization and delivery of these benefits. As originally written, Medicare instructed the federal government to cover any "reasonable costs" billed by hospitals and doctors. The public sector, therefore, was obliged to participate in the private market for health care, even though it had little influence in controlling costs.

The steep increase in the cost of health care and the explosion of public expenditures for health in the United States led to a shift in the focus of health reform, from improving access to health insurance to controlling the costs of health care. The Nixon administration's program for group-based health insurance was unsuccessful, although it did encourage the proliferation of health maintenance organizations (HMOs) in the United States and was considered the forerunner of "managed care" proposals (Brown 1983). Throughout the 1970s, Congressional Democrats attempted to link access and cost concerns with renewed demands for national health insurance, but the enduring divisions within the Democratic Party on the issue, the hostility of the Republican opposition, and the persistent resistance of provider groups precluded such reform initiatives (Marmor 1983).

The widespread reluctance to embark on new spending for entitlement programs and the neoconservative backlash pushed national health insurance out of the spotlight in the 1980s. At this point, reforming health care meant reducing federal expenditures, particularly spending on entitlement programs such as Medicare and Medicaid. Federal payments for Medicaid programs were substantially reduced, forcing states to modify their benefits and eligibility criteria. Medicare was a more difficult target, since it enjoyed widespread bipartisan support, bolstered by a large and politically influential clientele group, the aged. Despite the free-market rhetoric of the administration, the focus of health reform shifted to the regulation of the market for health services by imposing limits on Medicare payments, most significantly through the replacement of reimbursement of "reasonable costs" with a prospective schedule of fees based on diagnostic-related groups (or DRGs) (Morone and Dunham 1985). In 1984 and 1986, freezes were imposed on Medicare reimbursements for physician fees. At the same time, private insurers began to impose greater restrictions on the type and extent of reimbursement they would cover. Ironically, American doctors, who had fought compulsory national health insurance on the grounds of physician autonomy, now found themselves increasingly regulated by insurers and more awash in paperwork and billing problems than their Canadian counterparts working within a public health insurance system.

By the late 1980s, as health expenditures continued to soar in the United States, cost concerns became inextricably related to questions of access to care. A major health initiative of this period, the 1988 Medicare Catastrophic Coverage Act, was designed to improve the access of the elderly to long-term care. The measure was repealed under pressure from the elderly, who objected to the self-financing of the program through premiums and increased personal income tax. The rise and fall of the Medicare Catastrophic Coverage Act provides insight into the difficulty of restricting health care in the United States. The passage of this bill reflected a bipartisan recognition of the linkage between problems of cost and access. However, its subsequent demise revealed the limits of incremental change and pointed toward the need for a more fundamental restructuring of the American health care system.

The retrenchment of federal financing of existing programs and the relative inaction in addressing problems of health care costs and access encouraged states to think about initiating their own health reform (Iglehart 1994). Until 1988, the only successful state-level health insurance model was that of Hawaii, which combined mandatory employer-based coverage with cost containment. By 1992, Massachusetts, Minnesota, Vermont, and Florida had enacted (though not yet implemented) health care legislation; Oregon also proposed the rationing of certain Medicaid benefits. Within the next year, several more states would act, while virtually every state legislature would consider some type of health reform proposal. This state-level activity bolstered confidence in the idea that a national health insurance system could develop from subnational initiatives, as it had in Canada, and that such initiatives could allow states to experiment with different types of reform, from managed care to single-payer plans. But the problems surrounding such action, and the difficulty of reaching consensus in state legislatures, highlighted the limits of state-led reform in the US in the absence of a clear federal policy direction.

In 1991, Democrat Harris Wofford's upset victory over former Attorney General Richard Thornburgh in the Pennsylvania Senate race revealed the emerging political stakes of health reform as a national issue on the domestic agenda. This also showed the depth of dissatisfaction among voters with the perceived inaction of the Bush administration on the issue. In a recession-racked economy, working Americans feared for their health benefits. These fears were intimately tied to concerns about the future viability of the American health care system. The hard-to-define but politically powerful American "middle class" seemed worried that their access to affordable health insurance was in jeopardy, and were apprehensive about the future of the health care system. The medical lobby began to raise concerns about the problems of access to care, in particular the burden of caring for the uninsured and the limits imposed on their practices by third-party insurers. Once a bulwark against government intervention, the American Medical Association now endorsed a "public-private partnership" that would guarantee universal access while preserving the freedom of the medical profession in the health care market. Big business, saddled with a major portion of the American health bill, was increasingly frustrated by the seemingly uncontrollable increase in health costs and became another unlikely proponent of government regulation (Martin 1993).

During the 1992 election campaign, health reform surged to the centre of the domestic political agenda in the United States. President Bush seemed incapable of allaying fears about the economic future of the country, and of devising a reasonable scenario for health care reform. By contrast, "health care crisis" became oft-repeated buzzwords of the successful Clinton campaign that, along with it's "the economy, stupid," captured the attention of a recession-weary public open to the bold rhetoric of change.

This rhetoric was in evidence on September 22, 1993, as President Clinton delivered an emotional plea to Congress about the urgent need for health care reform in the United States. Clinton's address reflected the powerful momentum of the health reform issue that had helped propel the Democratic Party to the White House. But, as with Truman and Kennedy before him, the forcefulness of his delivery also reflected the offensive strategy he needed to implement in order to raise public engagement and face the substantial open hostility of powerful lobbies and their Congressional allies (for an account of this period, see Hacker 1997; Skocpol 1996).

As the Clinton administration began to tackle the health reform issue through a task force chaired by the First Lady, Hillary Clinton, several potential alternatives were already being discussed in policy circles. Interest in the Canadian health care system and its ability to balance cost control and access to care led to suggestions for a single-payer government-financed health insurance system supported by influential health care experts, consumer lobby groups, union organizations, and progressive Democrats. At the other extreme were Republican proposals for tax credits, vouchers, and medical savings accounts. In between were suggestions for expanding the existing Medicare model to other groups in society, as well as a number of variations on mandating employer health insurance.

And so, Canada had become an unwitting player in the debate over health reform in the United States. The Canadian model was not an unfamiliar one to Americans, and proponents of national health insurance had taken an interest in the Canadian experience since the 1970s (see Andreopoulos 1975). Canada was attracting renewed attention as the debate for health reform heated up in the 1990s, and as the search for solutions focused on issues of cost and access. As would be the case in 2008, the Canadian system figured prominently in the scenarios for health care reform in the United States, alternatively portrayed as a familiar model that could overcome "disinformation" about public medicine, or as the "cure worse than the disease."

Advocates of the Canadian model pointed out that a single-payer system could reap substantial savings in the overall costs of health care, while at the same time guarantee universal access to comprehensive benefits. A widely cited 1991 report for the United States General Accounting Office projected that such an arrangement could save the United States billions of dollars (GAO 1991). Other studies went further, suggesting cost savings on administrative waste (Woolhandler and Himmelstein 1991). These savings were accrued through simplified billing systems, global budgets, and negotiated fee schedules.

For their part, detractors pounced on Canadian health care as a straw man to demonstrate the impossibility of a single-payer system (see Maioni 1994). Their alternative estimates showed that total costs could actually increase under a Canadian-style system, and, ominously, that beyond the question of costs was a more fundamental question about the inevitable trade-off between quality and access. Stories abounded associating the rationing of health care and queuing for treatment with arbitrary government control of health resources and the constraints this imposed on freedom of choice. Media coverage in the US increasingly focused on Canada's perceived shortage of high-technology equipment, waiting lists for surgery, and overcrowding in hospitals. In addition, the Canadian medical community was accused of freeloading off the United States for high-quality research, innovative procedures, and medical technology. In a rebound effect, these arguments were quickly imported by conservative voices on the north side of the border.

For a brief moment in the debate over health reform in the 1990s, several influential voices continued to endorse the Canadian model, substantial numbers of Democrats in the House of Representatives supported a single-payer health insurance bill, and single-payer initiatives began to be discussed at the state level. Nevertheless, it was apparent that any variation on the Canadian model would not be part of the administration's reform package. In presenting his legislative proposals for health reform in 1993, President Clinton categorically rejected the single-payer model on the grounds that it was impractical and would require a massive influx of new taxes. Clinton and his administration continued to stress that their reform proposals for guaranteed private insurance represented a feasible, market-based alternative to a government-run single-payer system.

In effect, the Clinton plan that emerged in 1993 represented a departure from the basic social insurance precedent of the existing Medicare program. Instead of expanding eligibility through Social Security, the emphasis was on expanding coverage through employer mandates, and a mechanism for cost control through "managed competition" in health insurance markets. Specifically, this meant government regulation of private insurers through the creation of regionally based "health alliances." Clinton's reform proposal thus embraced government intervention in health care while retaining the legitimacy of private markets in health insurance.

But the Clinton compromise aimed at forging a middle path through the public regulation of health insurance markets failed to rally enough support from proponents of health reform. At the same time, these reforms also faced considerable opposition from powerful groups with vested interests in maintaining the profitable private health care system. Insurance lobbies, in particular, waged effective public campaigns against the Clinton proposals and, more broadly, against government involvement in health care. Within Congress, the administration faced opposition not only from Republican opponents but also from within the Democratic caucus. The opposition, interestingly, came from both directions. At one end, the proposals were criticized by those who wanted a more comprehensive and universal model; on the other, from the party's more fiscally conservative wing. There was widespread public confusion over the details of the president's health plan, compounded by the spectacle of political warfare between Congress and the administration, and the all-out efforts of powerful lobbies, especially the insurance industry. The bill finally died an ignoble bipartisan death, killed as much by Democratic fears as by Republican fear-mongering.

In the wake of the collapse of Clinton's health care reform, the Republican party launched an "anti-government" message that attacked the basic premise of public involvement in social programs and set the stage for the historic sweep of Congress in 1994 (Skocpol 1996). With control of the legislative agenda in the hands of a new breed of right-wing activists, national health insurance was gone for good. Nevertheless, the relentless pressure of cost and access concerns did not go away.

In fact, some of the initiatives that did move forward under Clinton would affect the shape of future health reform. The most important of these was welfare reform in 1996, which was followed by a major expansion of Medicaid through the Children's Health Insurance Program. Introduced through bipartisan sponsorship in the Senate—namely, Democratic liberal Ted Kennedy and Republican conservative Orrin Hatch—the measure dedicated federal funding to state programs that covered children in low-income families but not eligible for welfare benefits.

Clinton's successor, George W. Bush, was not interested in carving out a domestic policy legacy, and certainly not one that had to do with health care. Still, he did sign into law the Medicare Modernization Act of 2003. This expanded the role of private health insurance in Medicare Part C by allowing Medicare beneficiaries to enroll in privately managed care plans. The new law was also designed to address an important gap in benefits by creating a new Medicare Part D program that offered enrollment into a multiplicity of private drug plans for outpatient prescriptions. But the partisan divide and the stakeholder lobbying over this measure were as keen as ever. Democrats in Congress were thwarted in their attempts to include guarantees for more affordable drug prices and a national formulary for drugs covered.

By the time Bush was winding down his second term in office, the same sentiment regarding the unfinished business of health reform that had plagued his father more than a decade earlier was still apparent. By 2005, health costs were soaring to almost 17 percent of GDP, and the numbers of uninsured rose to over 45 million by 2005, one in six Americans (Bodenheimer and Grumbach 2012).

How the US is Different in Health Care

Despite differences in political culture or in the timing of welfare state development among the advanced industrialized countries, there seems to be a widespread consensus about the "right" to health care, and the need for compulsion and regulation by government to guarantee this right. Governments in Canada and other industrialized countries have sought to do so by openly confronting health care providers through the political process and treating health care as a public good. Until recently, the United States was the exception to this rule.

For all that, Canada and the United States have many similarities in their health care landscapes. Solo physician practice, private fee-for-service care, the dominance of voluntary hospitals, charity care based on philanthropic, religious, or community care, and direct government involvement limited to public health services were essential characteristics of both countries until midcentury. In both Canada and the United States, medical associations developed out of a desire to strengthen the monopoly of professional physicians and to regulate the practice of medicine. Since the 1910s, medical education on both sides of the border has retained important linkages, accreditation of medical schools falls under the same agencies, and licensing of physicians remains reciprocal across states and provinces. Even today, the delivery of health care in the two countries retains striking similarities. Voluntary, non-profit hospitals dominate the health sector in both countries. The majority of physician services are still based on private practice and fee-for-service remuneration. There are, however, major differences in the costs and financing of health benefits, and in the structure of, and coverage provided by, government-funded health insurance.

The American health insurance system is complex and difficult to describe (the description below relies on Bodenheimer and Grumbach 2012). The majority of Americans rely on employer-based benefits or private insurance coverage. But there is a significant portion of the health care economy that is centred on publicly funded health care. Over 40 percent of Americans—including veterans and military personnel, the elderly, disabled, and poor—enjoy some form of public coverage. For these groups, the major government programs remain Medicare and Medicaid. The latter is a federal-state social assistance program based on a means test that reimburses hospital and physicians that care for the 48 million Americans, including families and children, who qualify. Administered by the states, Medicaid plans are jointly financed by federal and state governments. In 1997, coverage was extended to eight million children in low-income families who would not otherwise be eligible in the form of the State Children's Health Insurance Programs (SCHIP), in which federal funds to help states cover children in poor families. Medicaid became the fastest-growing social program in the US after 1997. In 2007, President Bush vetoed a bill to increase federal contributions to SCHIP even though the measure enjoyed bipartisan support; one of President Obama's first acts in office in 2009 was to sign the bill to reauthorize and expand SCHIP.

Medicare enrolls 48 million elderly or disabled Americans eligible for social security benefits under US law. Medicare Part A works like a social insurance system and covers hospital benefits directly paid by the federal government and financed by compulsory payroll contributions. Medicare Part B offers supplementary medical insurance for physician care, financed through monthly premiums and heavily subsidized by Medicare as a whole. However, Medicare beneficiaries are responsible for paying substantial deductibles and co-insurance charges. Hospital care under Part A is limited to 60 days full coverage and up to 180 days of partial coverage of in-patient costs, plus 100 days of nursing home care per episode of illness, after deductibles. Part B covers 80 percent of approved medical care charges; patients are responsible for the remaining 20 percent plus deductibles. Many Medicare beneficiaries opt for supplementary medigap policies to cover the high costs of out-of-pocket expenditures, and some of that pressure was addressed by the so-called Medicare Part C, or Medicare Advantage, which allows individuals to join group plans. Finally, the most recent Medicare Part D offers prescription drug coverage insurance through a system of premiums, deductibles, and co-payments; initially, however, there was a significant gap, known as the "donut hole," which left beneficiaries with chronic conditions subject to a period of significant lack of coverage.

Because of the complexity and permeability of the employer-based American health insurance system, the number of uninsured people in the US has been a political issue for decades. Most recent estimates peg this number at about 50 million Americans not covered by any form of insurance, either private or public. In addition, millions more are considered "underinsured"—that is, insured for only part of their potential total health bill.

Congressional responses to the issue have included the Consolidated Omnibus Budget Reconciliations Act reforms of 1985. A clause in the omnibus budget package obliged employers to offer to extend health insurance benefits to workers who lose their jobs for a maximum of 18 months and with no obligation for employers to pay part of the premiums. In 1986, Congress passed the Emergency Medical Treatment and Active Labor Act (EMTALA), also known as the patient "anti-dumping" law. This piece of legislation obliges hospital emergency rooms to screen and stabilize patients who arrive on their doorstep, regardless of ability to pay.

The patchwork nature of US health insurance is not the system's only exceptionalism; so, too, are the costs associated with health care services. In 1960, health expenditures in the US represented just over 5 percent of GDP—a figure comparable to many countries, and almost identical to Canada. By 1975, health expenditures in the US rose to 8 percent, and by 1990 the gap between the US and others had widened considerably, to over 12 percent. As it hovers at 18 percent of GDP today, cost control and coverage for the uninsured have become the twin priority issues of health reform in the US (Maioni 2014).

Economists suggest that there are several reasons for these cost differences. First among them is the structure of the US economy, in particular a higher GDP per capita overall. This affects both the costs of health care services and the ability to pay for them. Prices for health care professionals, infrastructure, equipment, technology, and prescription drugs tend to be much higher in the US than elsewhere. The market power of the "supply side" of health care (doctors, hospitals, and pharmaceutical companies) has exacerbated the situation. Because of the multiple payers and purchasers of health care in the US, costs are not controlled to the same extent as in countries where governments have a larger role to play in purchasing health care services, negotiating with providers, regulating health care budgets, and rationing access to care. The complexities in payment for both private and public spending in the US have been shown to have an impact on costs as well, through higher administrative overhead. Others have pointed to the impact of malpractice litigation and the practice of "defensive medicine."

Recent Health Reform Strategies

Despite the divisive political and partisan battles over health reform in the US, as a rule, the Democrats favor reform to expand coverage subsidized by government and employers, while the Republicans favor free-market, consumer-based approaches. And these were indeed the essential fault lines in the most recent round of health reform in the US.

Early on in the 2008 primary campaign, Barack Obama sought to distinguish and distance himself from his main rival, Hillary Clinton. His campaign made children the priority, with education as the bedrock of his vision. As it emerged, his position on health care was to advocate subsidies and tax credits to help the uninsured acquire coverage, while at the same time requiring that all children have health insurance. Like most other Democrats, the men and women on Obama's policy team were confident that the money for these initiatives could be found by rolling back President Bush's tax cuts for higher-income households. But throughout the primary season, Obama shied away from the idea of forcing people to purchase insurance they might not be able to afford.

Hillary Clinton, in contrast, made health care the central point of her political platform from the beginning, and made no bones about where she stood on health reform. In so doing, she was handling a double-edged political sword. As First Lady, she had been in charge of the ill-fated health task force whose reform efforts failed miserably in Congress. But while the central component of the Clintons' earlier approach was the idea of employer mandates, by 2008, the focus had changed. Now, Hillary Clinton's approach would involve individual mandates that would require everyone to purchase health insurance.

Ironically, the idea of individual mandates—which recognized the need for legal obligation to compel universal coverage—was bolstered by the demonstration effect of a state-led initiative under Republican Governor Mitt Romney. The Massachusetts Health Care Reform Plan of 2006 required state residents to carry health insurance, and forced employers to offer coverage to their workers or pay an assessment fee. This effort was directly aimed at reducing the number of uninsured and lowering the cost drain on the state's health care system. As a presidential hopeful, however, Romney refused to support a nationwide expansion of this model.

Despite the heavy attention on the economy and the war in Iraq during the party conventions, health care was still on voter's minds across the US as middle-class issues took the forefront in the 2008 campaign. Unlike previous recent campaigns in which Medicare had been a central feature, health care this time around became an issue of personal economic import, part of the "pocketbook" issues that tend to preoccupy voters in tense economic times.

Obama's twin framing of health care reform in terms of both access and cost control was a deft strategy to capture the urgency of the issue in the context of the economic crisis. It was also a way to court crucial support from both Democrats and Republicans in the Congress. The other adroit move was to open up policy discussions and engage with stakeholders, instead of opting for the relatively closed approach that doomed Hillary

Clinton's 1993 task force. Obama also tried to distance himself from Bill Clinton's top-down approach by asking Congress to take the lead in writing the legislation. But without a central script, Democrats began to devise competing strategies, while Republicans and their allies, sensing a policy vacuum and a political opportunity, went to work in redefining health care reform—and the President himself—in the most negative terms possible.

By the time Obama took his place in the parade of presidents who have made health care reform addresses to the Congress, his message had firmed up considerably: "I am not the first president to take up this cause, but I am determined to be the last" (Obama 2009). Despite the eloquence of language and passion of delivery, Obama's insistence on the basic elements of reform—insurance regulation, cost control measures, and individual mandates—was crowded out by the deep divisions over the so-called public option. For supporters, the public option is essential because it would serve as a last-resort option for those who could not otherwise find or afford insurance coverage. For detractors, it represents (yet again) a wedge of socialized medicine on the one hand, and unfair competition on the other.

Once again, Canada entered the health care reform debate in the US, but this time the stakes and the situation had changed. In 1993, the single-payer model had been used as evidence by both opponents and supporters of health reform; in 2009, the targets were much more precise and the coverage of Canada almost entirely negative. Parallels were drawn between the public option and the deficiencies of the Canadian public insurance systems, while infamous ads featuring a "survivor" of the Canadian system and talk radio debates over "death panels" tried to illustrate the havoc that could be wreaked by constraining consumer choice and access. Although these new attacks were as misleading as their predecessors, they resonated more powerfully because the debate over health care on this side of the border had itself changed, leading to a noticeable erosion of confidence among some Canadians.

The Patient Protection and Affordable Care Act

What emerged from the Obama administration was a remarkable piece of legislation: remarkable in that it survived the travails of the Congress, despite considerable skepticism by many Democrats and overt hostility in Republican ranks; and remarkable also in that, despite its limitations in cost control and the failure of a public option, it represented a piece of legislation that would have an effect on health care for every American, insured or not.

The Patient Protection and Affordable Care Act (commonly referred to as the ACA) is, in many respects, an attempt to reform the way that insurers do business in the health field. While state regulations about insurance predate the ACA, the federal government has now taken on the task of reading the riot act to the insurance industry. Insurance practices such as rescission of coverage, lifetime limits on coverage, or denial of coverage based on pre-existing conditions will now be subject to federal law. A cap on co-payments and out-of-pocket payments also sent a warning signal about cost control to insurers and relief to those insured.

The ACA also took aim at two of the most pressing gaps in Medicare coverage: drug benefits and primary care. The passage of Medicare Part D had remained a thorn in many Democrats' sides, since they considered the coverage inadequate. Nowhere was this more evident than in the so-called donut hole—where beneficiaries found themselves once they reached the initial drug coverage limit but before they became eligible for catastrophic drug coverage. The ACA was designed to close that hole by offering discounts on the cost of brand name drugs to people in that situation. In addition, Medicare will now cover the costs of annual checkups, eliminate co-payments for preventive services, and provide financial incentives to primary care physicians taking on Medicare patients.

Of course, the ACA's historic breakthrough was to directly address the problem of the uninsured in the US. A federal insurance mandate was accompanied by a system of federal subsidies for state insurance exchanges that were directed to regulate insurance offerings so that the mandate could be implemented effectively. Subsidies were also provided to small business owners so they could offer affordable coverage to employees. And, for the first time since its creation, Medicaid has now been extended to eligible single adults (and is not limited to family households, as in the past).

Although the ACA, passed in March 2010, was to be implemented over a number of years (the mandate, for example, was set to come into effect in 2014), legal challenges were mounted almost immediately in federal courts around the US. For example, a Virginia federal court invalidated the insurance mandate of the law; a Florida federal court ruled that this unconstitutionality required the invalidation of the entire law. Given the political stakes at hand, the Supreme Court took on the case with alacrity, hearing arguments in March 2012. Three crucial questions were asked. First, does the US Commerce Clause grant Congress the power to impose a mandate (by requiring state residents to maintain a minimum level of health insurance or pay a tax penalty)? Second, can the ACA survive if the individual mandate does not? And third, did Congress violate principles of federalism by pressuring states to change their eligibility criteria by threatening to withhold federal funding under Medicaid? The Court was divided in its deliberations, even though the major provisions of the ACA held. The Court ruled that the federal government could not force individuals to purchase insurance (although it could impose a tax penalty if they did not), and it could not force states to set up health exchanges nor to expand their Medicaid systems.

It is estimated that the new legislation will extend insurance coverage to 32 million uninsured Americans, with a price tag of over $900 billion (Bodenheimer and Grumbach 2012). Coverage is now mandated (with health insurance exchanges and subsidies making it easier to find affordable insurance packages), regulation of insurers has been tightened, Medicare gaps have been addressed, and access to Medicaid considerably expanded. But there is no public option or opening toward "national" health insurance of the Canadian or European kind.

In the end, the passage of the Patient Protection and Affordable Care Act of 2010 was both a political coup and a hard-won compromise, reflecting not only active bipartisan cleavages (not a single Republican in Congress voted in favour) but also the nature of deeply divided public opinion.

Whither National Health Insurance?

During this partisan war over health reform, Canada again became a poster child for the right in Washington and across the US. The most virulent critics of reform again raised the spectre of "Canadian-style" health care.

And yet, there is no way that the ACA could be mistaken for a single-payer system. The new legislation keeps the US's traditional multi-payer structure in place, while adding another layer through the introduction of health care exchanges for the uninsured. In so doing, the ACA reinforces what Ted Marmor has referred to as the "five Americas" of health care that involve a "patchwork" of the different coverage and payment scenarios sketched out above: employer-based care, Medicare, Medicaid, EMTALA, and the Veteran's Administration (Marmor and Wendt 2010).

This does not resemble equal universal coverage of the kind Canadians would recognize in their provincial health plans. In the US, access to care will still depend on the kind of insurance Americans can buy, or the entitlement program to which they belong, only now Americans will be compelled by federal law to prove that coverage or face a tax penalty. The ACA does try to make this coverage more affordable and to even the playing field in its provisions for insurance reform. But the new law reinforces the principle that access to care depends on what you can afford or what you are entitled to, not what you actually need. Even the health insurance exchanges offer premiums based on age, health, income, and on whether you opt for bronze, silver, gold, or platinum coverage.

Nor has the ACA ended up creating "national" health insurance, or the situation in which Canadians can at least aspire to coverage for a comprehensive range of services, no matter where they live. And in which, despite the ebb and flow of federal largesse to the provinces, both levels of government are seen to have roles and responsibilities in this policy area. As we have seen, federalism provides a complex policy environment for health care matters in Canada; in the US, however, federalism feeds into an even more fractious political environment. The implementation of the ACA will likely exacerbate the situation, and leave even more divisions and discrepancies in health care access and coverage from state to state.

And, finally, even if the Affordable Care Act will make health care more affordable for some Americans, it does not have the means to make health care more affordable for the US government. The new law has dozens of provisions, including a review of Medicare reimbursement and the expansion of accountable care organizations to reward cost-effective care. But it doesn't grapple in a systematic fashion with the overall inefficiencies in health care financing, the administrative burden of multiple payers, providers, and plans, and the cost pressures of defensive medicine. As we well know, paying for health services is a huge financial concern for Canadian governments, but there is the underlying requirement that all taxpayers contribute to make this happen, and governments have at their disposal at least some cost containment measures that remain difficult, if not impossible, in the current American context.

Despite the hyperbole, then, the Affordable Care Act did little to change the essential differences between the two health care systems. In fact, its most enduring impact may be to "lock in" the private insurance system of access to care in the US, rather than moving toward anything like national health insurance.

Comparing Canada and Europe

A French adage suggests, *quand je me regarde, je me désole, mais quand je me compare, je me console* ("when I look at myself, I am sad; when I compare myself, I am glad"). Can the same be said of Canada's health care system?

Comparative analysis informs us about how and why countries faced with similar challenges or problems might nevertheless end up with different choices when it comes to solutions (Klein and Marmor 2012). Even though countries might resemble one another or aspire to similar goals— for example, universality in health care coverage—they might have different approaches and routes to these objectives. In health care reform, much of that difference has to do with the political, economic, and social context on the ground.

As we have seen, the United States always looms large as a comparator for Canadians. It makes sense, given the close cultural, economic, and social linkages between the two countries, and it also follows the logic of comparative analysis as well. Both countries are considered liberal welfare states (Esping-Andersen 1990), and they remain both very similar to each other (in terms of delivery of care, and professional practice) and very different (in terms of financing and insurance).

Nevertheless, in the patterns of health care spending and public health plans, many European countries also provide a useful comparison and contrast. For some, the European experience offers a good reminder of the underlying values of universal coverage and the power of regulatory frameworks (Marmor, Okma, and Latham 2006); for others it been touted as an example of the way in which public and private health care systems can co-exist (Simpson 2012).

In this chapter, we take a look at where Canada "fits" among a peer group of industrialized countries and then look in more depth at two cases—Britain and Germany—to further explore the notion of lessons from European cases.

The Comparative Context

As the most reliable cross-national surveys of health care make plain, there is no systematic leader in performance (Schoen et al. 2007). This is important to keep in mind when comparing health care systems. Indeed, the main similarity among different health systems across the industrialized world is the extent to which they need to face both organizational and financial challenges. Demographic pressures, cost and access concerns, changing medical practice, technological changes, coordination and integration of care: all of these are features of policy discussions not only in Canadian health systems but the world over.

While the United States is an outlier with regard to any possible measure associated with regulation, access, and spending in health care, Canada falls more readily into the pattern of European and other industrialized nations. And yet, even here, there are idiosyncrasies that point to a unique Canadian model.

Take health care spending, for example. With 11 percent of GDP devoted to health, Canada definitely falls into the "big spender" category along with some of its European counterparts, even though all of these countries spend considerably less than the United States. Given the reinvestment in health care spending over the past decade, Canada's rate of spending growth has been higher, although no other country experienced the kind of slash-and-burn approach to public funding that Canada did in the 1990s.

Instead, many European governments chose to experiment with mixing the financing options in the health care sectors, from allowing parallel private-delivery systems to permitting individual co-payments for patients and introducing internal markets to generate competition among providers.

Still, in many ways that have been pointed out in previous chapters, Canada has its own "mixed" system. Public health insurance plans are universal in their eligibility and offer equal access to care, resolutely enshrined in the principle of "first-dollar" coverage: all the services covered in provincial health plans, whether accessed in a hospital or through a physician—are covered at 100 percent of the cost. And yet the basket of services outside this definition of care is not as extensive as in other countries, where some forms of nominal co-payment may be in place. Almost 30 percent of total health care spending in Canada is non-public, a much higher proportion than in most industrialized countries, with the exception of the US. Part of this discrepancy comes from the exclusion of big-ticket items, especially prescription drugs, from provincial public plans.

Canada is also unique in its approach to the balance between public and private provision of financing of health care services. The much-touted compromise between "public payment, private delivery" (Naylor 1986) allows considerable autonomy for medical practitioners in maintaining a fee-for-service practice, but it also sets up a tighter wall between public and private payment. For example, physicians cannot "double-dip" through the extra billing of public-pay patients or through simultaneously taking on private-pay patients, something that is often tolerated in other health care systems. Moreover, the ability to expand private-pay alternatives is constricted by rules that make it difficult for private insurers to offer coverage of any publicly insured service, a condition that was challenged in the courts in Quebec. Likewise, the financing of Canadian hospitals is also somewhat unique: fee-for-service physicians co-existing with rigid global budgets, instead of the mix of payment features that often come into play elsewhere.

Even the development of government involvement in the health care sector renders Canada's experience unique. In comparison to Europe, Canada was a latecomer in implementing public hospital and medical insurance in the 1950s and 1960s. As in the US, private insurance coverage, mainly employer-based, dominated until then. By contrast, most European countries inaugurated health insurance in the immediate postwar era, often building from pre-existing sickness insurance practices and programs.

Beyond timing, one of the most obvious differences between the Canadian and European systems is the extensive role of subnational governments—from the origins of the public model in Saskatchewan to the enduring responsibilities of provincial governments in the health care sector. There is an obvious contrast with unitary countries, such as the UK and France, where central governments are in the driver's seat for much of the administrative structure for health services financing and delivery. But even in other federal countries, such as Australia and Germany, for example, both levels of government share responsibility for health care, while the central government retains the principal regulatory powers.

Even in the sense of imposing "norms," Canada has developed its own way of doing things. Health care is not a right enshrined in any constitutional sense, as it is in some European cases, nor is public provision and financing an ironclad responsibility for governments to take on. And yet, most Canadians feel very strongly about their health care system, its strengths and weaknesses, and have come to internalize the sense of obligation that governments have in ensuring access to comprehensive and timely care.

A Tale of Two Models

A good starting point to understand European experiences in health care would be to consider how they developed in very different contexts. As we've learned, Canada's system is referred to as a single-payer model, because public money flows in and out of a single "tap"—the provincial and territorial health plans.

In the European context, there are two main models. One adopts social insurance financing (e.g., Germany, France, Netherlands) the other tends toward a national health "service" or system (e.g., UK, Sweden, Italy). Scholars often categorize these approaches by distinguishing between "Bismarckian" and "Beveridge" models (Fierlbeck 2011; Marmor, Freeman, and Okma 2009).

The first set—the Bismarckian models—are characterized by social insurance, which means that insurance coverage is compulsory for all workers in the country. Moreover, everyone must contribute into a designated fund (this is also the basis for Medicare in the US), usually based on income, with government supplements for those not in the labour market (Carrin and James 2005).

The Beveridge model, meanwhile, developed in post-World War II Britain, with a different logic based on universal coverage and public financing in which the general revenues of the state were used to fund more centralized health care systems. This is the basis for the British National Health Service, as well as the Swedish and Italian health care systems.

Social insurance for workers in Germany

Not surprisingly, the first social insurance system was introduced in Germany in the late 19th century, a period of particularly acute tension between the growing power of labour organizations and social democratic parties on the one hand, and the imperial state under the administration of Chancellor Otto von Bismarck on the other (Manow 1997). The 1883 Health Insurance Law was designed to cover workers—and co-opt them, too—through federal social insurance by occupational group, beginning with certain blue-collar workers. The German model became the basis for several state-led initiatives during the progressive era in the US; these were ill-fated, however, drowned out by the anti-German sentiment of World War I.

Over time, all sectors of the German work force were covered by these sickness funds, which stretched into over a thousand occupational and regional groups. This process accelerated after World War II in West Germany, while East Germany's health system turned to a state-controlled model, with publicly owned polyclinics and salaried physicians. With reunification in the 1990s, the sickness fund model of social insurance was extended across the whole country (Manow 1997). By the early 2000s, it became apparent that the health care delivery system was under intense cost pressures. Still, the overwhelming popularity of the system limited the policy choices available to pro-market Chancellor Angela Merkel after 2006, transforming what had initially been major reform into a series of compromise measures that included lowering the income needed to opt out of the sickness funds, and increasing payroll tax contributions.

In Germany today, therefore, health insurance is tied to employment status, a different calculation than in Canada. But the compulsory nature of the system and heavy public regulation means that almost 90 percent of the German population is covered for health care through a choice of sickness funds (today, there are 250 such funds, and they are no longer based on occupation). The remaining population (civil servants and higher-income Germans) can opt out to purchase private insurance. Unlike general-revenue financing for provincial and territorial plans in Canada, these German sickness funds are based on mandated payroll taxes shared by employers and employees to cover workers and their dependents. The federal government covers the unemployed through an earmarked social fund.

All of these funds are considered not for profit and are tightly regulated by the federal government. And while there is competition for subscribers among these plans, they all have to abide by the same fee schedules and hospital prices that are negotiated on a Lander (state) basis. So, as in Canada, subnational governance is importance, but unlike the Canadian experience—in which separate bargaining takes place with different components of the health care system in each province at different times—in Germany, state governments compel representatives of physicians and hospital associations to meet on a regular basis around the same table to arrive at compromises on fees and pricing through a "concerted action" process. And while drug manufacturers are free to set their own wholesale prices, the federal government regulates retail pricing, while the German practice of reference pricing means that patients are covered for pharmaceuticals only if they choose the lower-cost option.

While the mechanism for health care financing differs (payroll taxes rather than general revenues), Germany resembles Canada in that the system offers universal coverage and is publicly financed. But as in other social insurance systems (like France, and especially Japan), patient choice is paramount, both in the provision of primary care and in hospital care. And, the German sickness funds tend to cover much more than provincial and territorial plans: in addition to outpatient and in-patient care, they cover dental care, optometry, and prescription drugs.

There are also similarities in the way physician care is delivered and paid for. Like their Canadian counterparts, physicians in Germany are paid on a fee-for-service basis for outpatient care, and Germans have a relatively free choice of providers through their sickness funds. This means that, as in Canada, payment and reimbursement are administratively streamlined. Still, there are two differences to point out. First, there are caps on physician payment, so after a certain level, reimbursement rates drop significantly. Second, there are now co-payments on physician care, but these are also regulated and relatively minor, to the tune of 10 euros for the first quarter of the year, with exemptions for children and pregnant women. In hospitals, the co-payment is 10 euros per day (for the first 28 days). Despite these co-pays, their reach is very limited, and only 13 percent of total health spending in Germany is out of pocket.

Most German physicians working in hospitals would be envious of their Canadian colleagues, since the German doctors are paid on a salaried basis, and not all that well, either, by comparison. Hospitals, too, have a different payment system. The Lander are responsible for the functioning of their hospitals, deciding on their responsibilities, and regulating the system of payment for in-patient care through diagnosis-related groups rather than global budgets, as is the case in Canada.

Overall, then, a social insurance system such as Germany's offers interesting insights for Canada, as some observers have commented on (e.g., Greb et al. 2008). Some of these shed light on what is working well in both countries: cost control in hospital settings, and the co-existence of public payment with private practice for outpatient care. Still, critics in both countries point to the need for better coordination of primary care (in Germany, financial incentives are now being introduced to improve this), and the need for better measures for hospital performance based on quality and efficiency, not just volume of care.

Another insight has to do with the fact that, in both countries, money does not change hands at the point of contact with the health care system. This has an enormous impact on rationalizing administrative costs and imposing a certain logic and order in the delivery of care. The co-payments that do exist in the German context—minor at best, and tightly regulated in all circumstances—can hardly be thought of as a panacea, the way some observers reckon in the Canadian context.

The other illusory panacea is the role of a "parallel" private system. This so-called private insurance system is mainly used in the same way as in Canada—for supplemental insurance for amenities such as medical devices and the like—and heavily regulated by the federal government. The ability of Germans to entirely opt out of the sickness fund system has increased in the past decade, as the income threshold to do so has lowered over time.

But the number of Germans who choose to do so remains limited because of the higher cost and actuarial considerations of the plans (e.g., age), and because of the stipulation that once you opt out you cannot opt back in.

Finally, the German example provides a compelling story about the role of federalism and health care. Both the Lander and the federal government loom large in the German health care system, regulating sickness funds and private insurers, setting prices, and forcing negotiation for cost control among the principal players. While the Lander remain important in the functioning of the hospital system and the negotiation process over prices, the federal government has a significant role in ensuring solidarity in health reform and the strict regulatory framework for the health care market.

The battle for health care in Britain

While the Bismarckian initiatives did not create much of a ripple in Canada, the British interpretation of the German model certainly did (Naylor 1986). In the early 20th century, a new breed of liberalism emerged in Britain, symbolized by the National Insurance Act of 1911, a contributory sickness and unemployment plan for British workers. General practitioners were required to provide medical care under capitated rates to these workers, which initially led to considerable division with the medical class— uneasiness echoed by Canadian doctors across the Atlantic.

While Britain's medical insurance program did not establish a precedent for any major Canadian initiatives, it did set the stage for state involvement in health care in Britain. Although unwieldy and incomplete, the popularity of the plan, combined with the effects of a battle-weary population in the wake of World War II, was such that the Labour Party was able to win office in 1945 on the promise of a much more extensive reform. Like the CCF in Saskatchewan in 1944, Britain's first left-wing government would make electoral history through health care.

The National Health Service, inaugurated in 1948, was based on the vision of William Beveridge, a former civil servant and social reformer who had inspired Leonard Marsh's report on postwar reconstruction in Canada. They key point of the Beveridge model was the concept of a social minimum as the responsibility of all members of society. Thus, the NHS was based on a universal plan for "free" health services to which every taxpayer had to contribute. Despite the stringent opposition of physicians, the NHS nationalized British hospitals and their staffs, and extended general practitioner capitation coverage to the entire population (Klein 2010).

For decades, the combination of compulsion and centralization effectively constrained costs and provided a rigid system of equal access to health care based on capitation for general practitioners and specialist care through hospitals, all financed by general revenues and free at the point of service. But a major criticism was that, by the 1980s, Britons were facing some of the longest waiting times for treatment in the industrialized world. The other major problem was conflict between the medical communities and government on payment for health services.

The Conservative Party under Margaret Thatcher proved to be more of a game-changer in health care than the Mulroney government in Canada. The proposals for alternative sources of financing and tax incentives for private insurance were scuttled, but the review of the NHS by Alan Enthoven in 1985 did lead to the introduction of "internal markets" for health services, a controversial measure that basically meant hospitals now had to compete for public-pay patients as a way of increasing efficiency in the system. But without new injections of money into the tightly budgeted system, quality of care still suffered.

Enter Tony Blair and the Third Way in the 1990s, promising to address shortages of doctors and nurses, set targets for waiting times, modify contracts for GPs and hospital consultants, and allow a regulated market for private health services. Primary care trusts, which coordinate care between doctors and other providers, became the main access points for patients, while independent "foundation trusts" were set up to allow some autonomy within the NHS.

Blair's reforms, heavily geared toward quality of care and patient empowerment, with heavy emphasis on targets and performance, were based on the principle of "payment by results," in which money followed the patient through the public system. In addition, the NHS decentralized into constituent parts (NHS England, NHS Scotland, NHS Wales), giving them considerable autonomy. Still, it is not quite a federal arrangement as in Canada, since Whitehall still controls the purse when it comes to funding.

All of this came at a price. Health professionals and the health care workforce were understandably fatigued by the pace of constant change, although physicians were arguably well compensated through the reforms. In addition, Blair was accused of "creeping privatization"—even from within his own party—for persisting with the initiatives to allow doctors to practice privately and for setting up "independent sector" treatment, breaching the wall between public and private payment that still remains intact in Canada. Waiting lists have been reduced, but, say critics, at the cost of coherence in the delivery of care, equality of access, and in big increases in overall health care spending. And the NHS reforms have turned out to be hugely expensive, even though some of them were considered necessary reinvestments in the health care sector, including the establishment of electronic patient records.

Historically speaking, health care systems in the Canadian provinces were inspired more by Beveridge than Bismarck. And, politically speaking, the discourse of postwar reconstruction in Canada was filtered through the lens of Beveridge's social welfare state; the CCF (and, later, NDP) agenda for health insurance and the Labour Party's NHS were initially denounced as red-scare socialism.

In practice, the main similarity between Britain and Canada on this front is that health care is financed through general revenues, and delivered free at the point of service through the public system. Yet there are persistent structural differences as well. For example, physician payment retained a fee-for-service basis across the provinces, a feature that did not prevail in the NHS model, and that continues to be a source of conflict between the state and professional groups in Britain. The capitation process that serves as the basis for delivery of care through general practitioners in Britain is another key difference. Combined with what seems to be a more logical path of stepwise access to care and a more comprehensive care package (that includes dental care and prescriptions for children, the elderly, and those with low income), many point to the NHS model as more effective for both promotion of health and control of costs.

Another area where there is considerable attention on British lessons for Canada is the way in which hospitals are financed, moving away from a total reliance on global budgets to adopting some of the mechanisms for internal markets and for money that follows the patient through the hospital sector.

More recently, however, it is the obsession with data and deliverables, and the changes in the relationship between public and private payment that have received the most attention in Britain (Klein 2013). Critics in Canada bemoan the lack of data on outcomes, targets, and quality of care, and they are correct in pointing to some obvious transparency issues about which patients—and taxpayers—need better information. Yet, the NHS also offers a sobering example of the challenges of the collection and dissemination of such massive amounts of data.

The growth of the private sector in medical care is also a point of contention. Patients who receive a referral from their general practitioner may wait for an NHS consultation or consult a specialist through private access. The specialist in question, however, may be working in a publicly funded hospital while also seeing patients on a private-pay basis. This is, as yet, not possible in Canada, since physicians may accept only one form of payment, either public or private. The rationale in the British case is that these private consultations free up the backlog of people waiting to see specialists; critics, however, point to the "perverse incentives" that may encourage specialists to maintain longer NHS waiting times for consultations, and the mixed-system queue-jumping that may occur as private-pay consultations lead to more rapid referrals back to an NHS hospital for treatment.

More recently, the Health and Social Care Act that came into effect in 2013 is showing the reach of discontent within the medical community and how, paradoxically, the financial and professional autonomy of physicians can be challenged by the lifting of regulation. Physicians in both Canada and Britain opted in to the public system—by coercion or choice, as it may be—and have since relied on the guarantee of patients and payments through their agreement to serve the public system. Now, the NHS will allow a different sort of commissioning of treatment through tender, in which private organizations can compete to win contracts for care, with the emphasis on payment by results. The impact on physicians is expected to be substantial, as they will now be faced with pressures that have more to do with cost-efficient care managed by private organizations, rather than care based on a broader conception of patient need and population health.

Comparative Reflections

For years, critics of Canada's health care system have lamented the absence of European lessons in the design of health care reform. Usually, these concerns have been framed in terms of the need for more efficiency and revenue options through private investment, delivery, and financing of health care services.

Indeed, the European cases have provided content for reports that have suggested we might do well to consider a different mix of private and public measures for spending and delivery of care, one that would allow us to move beyond the zero-sum game that is often portrayed. In his 2002 health reform report, Senator Michael Kirby took similar inspiration from European cases to suggest that there might be a better mix of public and private delivery. Even the Supreme Court, in the narrow majority ruling on *Chaoulli v. Quebec* in 2005, referred to comparative evidence that such reform is necessary. On the provincial scene, Premier Gordon Campbell took a modern-day grand tour of European health care systems to examine the potential of their initiatives for British Columbia. And Claude Castonguay, the father of Quebec's health care system, returned to European examples in his recent report for the Quebec government, emphasizing the need for increased private investment in infrastructure and technology and the development of new private revenue streams and insurance models as the only way to salvage health care financing.

Certainly, Canada is not alone in the challenges it faces. Health care is rapidly becoming the most expensive of social programs the world over, and one in which the complexities of expanding needs, rising expectations, and new technologies are reshaping the policy agenda. Comparative experiences may indeed offer some insights into how European countries are facing these challenges.

Still, the comparative vignettes in this chapter show that shopping abroad for ready-made solutions is a fool's errand. The German and British cases offer some interesting and possibly enlightening points of comparison about the structure of the health care system, the role of parties and political institutions, and the unfolding of history across countries. And most comparative observers recognize that a careful reading of the past and present in European health care reform reveals the complexity and controversial nature of this policy area. The point is that a comparative perspective can shed light on the impact of specific reforms in particular circumstances, or on the general direction of reform in relation to that country's longer health policy trajectory. But these experiences remain rooted in distinctive and delimited contexts, making it difficult to pick and choose among the pack, or even to conclude that the impact over there may be the same over here.

Instead, it would seem that these reflections offer what comparative analysis is designed to do: offer insights into the similarities and differences across past experiences and future challenges. The first such insight would be to scuttle the perception that the funding of health care in Canada is somehow an aberration in the universe of cases. Like the vast majority of European countries, Canada offers to its legal residents sure and safe access to health care. It does so by compelling patients to share in the cost of care—in the Canadian case, through paying general taxes, not through fees and direct payment—and by compelling providers to play in the system, through a mix of regulation and financial incentives.

The mix of revenues is also evident by comparison. In Canada, the mix is determined by the type of service: medical and historical services are financed publicly; prescription drugs, dental, and other types of care are provided through private payment, either out of pocket or through supplementary insurance. Germany chooses a different type of mix, so too does Britain, but in both cases there is a mix—something that, arguably, already exists in the Canadian case.

Another feature regarding the funding of the Canadian system revealed through comparison is this country's unique blend of fee-for-service payment for physicians and global budgets for hospitals, a blend that differs from the payment mechanisms for providers in Germany and Britain but one that, apart from the more radical measures of the 2013 NHS reforms, is within the realm of how European countries deal with payment for care.

Second, the comparative cases shed some light on the costs of health care reform: there are, indeed, winners and losers or, to use a more discreet metaphor, health policy is a game of compromise and cost-sharing. Sometimes these costs are borne by patients, other times by providers, but usually it is a mix of the two. Still, it is important to realize that changing the nature of funding, payment, or access can have more portentous costs in terms of both equity and access. And there is really no conclusive evidence from the European experience to suggest that broadening alternative funding and delivery mechanisms actually provides more cost-efficient or better quality services, or improved distribution of health care resources or care. Governments may need to be much more upfront about the need for trade-offs and choices in the health care sector, but they cannot devolve themselves of responsibilities and expect only good news to prevail.

A third insight is that to make any type of public system work, regulation is the key. The German case shows this perhaps best, through the traditional corporatist bargaining structure that permeates the range of fees payment across the health care sector. In Britain, heavy public regulation had considerable cost-containment power in the past, but both positive and negative impacts on the organization and delivery of care. Many of the criticisms of the new health legislation, however, suggest that widening of the commissioning of health care services will lead to even more complex and heavy regulation and bureaucracy, not less.

And finally, in each of these countries—one federal, the other unitary; one Bismarkian, the other a Beveridge model—an important aspect of the health care system has been leadership from national governments. In this case, Canada is an interesting outlier, indeed. On paper, the subnational units in Canada have virtually full competence over the delivery and funding of publicly financed health care services, which is certainly not the situation in the majority of European cases, nor in the two models surveyed in this chapter.

In practice, of course, federal governments did take a leadership role in health care reform across the decades, but that role was usually about funding and dissemination, not necessarily about innovation or creativity. And while we have a high level of symmetry between the provinces and territories on the values and functioning of health care, the pan-Canadian coordination remains relatively thin in comparison to our European counterparts.

While this can be seen as something to celebrate (as an opportunity for subnational autonomy), as we shall see in the next chapter, and even a necessity for a population so diverse across a territory so vast, it may also mean that the potential for transformative change is always just beyond our horizon.

Chapter 6

Provincial Snapshots

It would be hard to overestimate the role of the provinces in health care, since the regulations that govern public health insurance across Canada are in the hands of provincial legislatures. We have already examined this impact in the delivery and financing of health care elsewhere in the book. But it bears returning to the actual content and evolution of health care services in the provinces to get a more comprehensive picture.

The best approach is to start with a few facts and figures. As has been already noted, there are provincial variations over health spending in Canada. For example, Canadian Institute for Health Information estimates for 2013 showed public health expenditures per capita average just below $4,000 for Canada as a whole, similar to the Ontario average; these vary from a high of over $5,300 in Newfoundland & Labrador, about $4,500 in Alberta and Saskatchewan, and only $3,500 in Quebec. Adding the territories into the mix brings further variations: the Yukon averages about $6,300, the NWT almost $7,000, while in Nunavut it's over $10,000 per capita. Private expenditures also show variations: Nova Scotia and New Brunswick have the highest such per capita expenditures, just over $2,000 each, while Quebec and Saskatchewan have the lowest, at $1,500 each. Similarly, there are slight differences in how much is spent in different sectors of the health economy. The province with the fastest-growing revenues, Alberta, is forecasted to have the highest expenditures in hospital spending and physician reimbursement; Quebec, meanwhile, has the lowest forecast. Despite these variations, one constant across the provinces is the extent to which health spending accounts for, on average, about 40 percent of total provincial budgets (CIHI 2013).

Provincial health plans share a similarity in that all medically necessary services are publicly insured, but there are nevertheless differences in organization, delivery, and access. For example, Quebec counts 18 regional health authorities (RHAs); Ontario now has 14. In 2012, Manitoba reduced the number of RHAs from 11 to 5; New Brunswick from 8 to 2. And in

Alberta, RHAs were abolished entirely in 2008. The ratio of physicians to population is relatively similar across the provinces, although that ratio is much lower in the territories, and particularly problematic for the provision of specialist care. The provinces have generally reduced wait times for a number of services since 2004, including cataract surgery and radiation treatment, but there is more variation for attaining benchmarks in hip and knee replacement surgeries.

The other point of difference is the use and cost of non-insured services, in particular outpatient pharmaceuticals. Quebec is the only province to have a universal pharmacare plan, which individuals can opt out of if they have employer-based coverage. Ontario offers a variety of supplemental plans, for seniors, low-income and long-term-care patients, as well as a program to cover the costs of medication for specific disease categories and, in some cases, new or experimental drugs. Most other provinces have some form of income and needs-based supplemental funding available, including British Columbia, Saskatchewan, Manitoba, and Newfoundland. Alberta and PEI also have "catastrophic" drug plans in effect.

An Overview of Provincial Health Care Systems

In order to understand the role of provinces in health policy, it's important to put these provincial snapshots in context. The rest of the chapter does so, first by reviewing the development of selected provincial and territorial systems, and then by looking in more depth at two provinces—namely, Saskatchewan and Quebec.

Health care politics in British Columbia

We start with the province of British Columbia, not only because it provides a geographical signpost (moving from west to east across Canada) but also because BC is a little-known pioneer in health care, having passed Canada's first public health insurance legislation in 1936. Then, as now, BC was a province with an activist labour movement and a strong leftist presence in the political arena. It was the first province to set up a Royal Commission on State Health Insurance in 1919, and it did so again in 1929 and 1932. During the Great Depression, the Liberal government of Duff Pattullo (who built his campaign on a New Deal-type platform for "Work and Wages") passed health insurance in 1936, despite the lack of financial guarantees from Ottawa and the collective opposition of both business leaders and the medical profession (Naylor 1986). In the end, despite the support of a majority of British Columbians, the plan failed to be implemented for precisely these reasons.

Nevertheless, British Columbia was the first province after Saskatchewan to enact hospital insurance, in 1948, predating the federal cost-sharing program. In 1965, the Social Credit government implemented the Medical Services Plan (MSP), before federal legislation once again. The MSP differed from the Saskatchewan initiative in that it was initially offered to those who did not have private insurance, and it required a premium-based payment. In 1996, BC's health laws were amalgamated into the Medicare Protection Act, which prohibited extra billing as a result of the Canada Health Act stipulations. Indeed, prior to this, BC had been one of the few provinces ever "charged" with violating CHA conditions.

The health care system in BC resembles that in the other provinces in terms of its scope and structure. However, residents are also charged a monthly premium based on income and family size, with subsidies for the lowest-income families. Non-insured services, such as dental care and optometry, are also provided for children in low-income families. In addition, BC has a pharmacare program that partially covers the cost of certain prescription drugs and medical supplies for specific patient populations. And, although the political debate remains fierce on wait times and access, almost 90 percent of BC residents report having a regular doctor, and only 13 percent report difficulty in accessing care (CIHI 2011).

Still, there are ongoing issues. The move toward decentralization was reversed, with five relatively autonomous health authorities taking the place of 52 health regions. One of the reasons was to better implement primary care reform, including BC's Primary Health Care Charter in 2007 and the Integrated Health Network in November 2008. Part of the impetus was to address chronic-care needs—an important concern, given BC's growing elderly population. Gordon Campbell's Liberal government also took a hard line with hospital unions in the 2000s, paving the way for the privatization of ancillary services (laundry, food, etc.), but not without strike action and concerns about the impact on infection rates in BC hospitals. And BC continues to be fertile ground for the proliferation of private health clinics and surgical facilities that offer a growing menu of services. The largest, the Cambie Surgery Centre in Vancouver, provides a full range of non-insured and insured services and has come under scrutiny for charging facility fees to patients. An injunction filed against the centre has been challenged in terms of the constitutionality of limiting consumer choice—and the court cases ahead will likely have an even greater impact on tracing that fine line between public and private services in Canada.

The case of Ontario

Historically speaking, Ontario played the role of dealmaker—and breaker—in health care reform. But while Premier George Drew shut down federal-provincial discussions on postwar reconstruction in 1945, a decade later Leslie Frost proved to be a decisive voice egging the federal government onward toward a cost-sharing program in hospital insurance (Taylor 1987). And, in 1959, the Ontario Hospital Services Plan was launched. As for medical insurance, the Progressive Conservative government did implement a plan in 1966, just before the federal legislation, but it was replaced in 1969 to correspond to the Medical Care Act, and adopted the moniker of OHIP (Ontario Health Insurance Plan) in 1972.

Since then, the legislation has been modified as a result of the extra-billing ban in the Canada Health Act. This led to a divisive confrontation in 1986 between the minority Liberal government and the Ontario Medical Association, reminding Canadians of the political stakes around publicly funded health insurance (Tuohy 1988). While the strike lasted less than a month, the repurcussions were significant. Ontario doctors continue to be politically mobilized and are a formidable bargaining group. Today, Ontario physicians tend to be among the best paid in Canada, and among the best paid professonals in the province, and fees have increased significantly over the last decade, including incentive fees for servicing remote areas or specific shortages in care.

As Ontario struggled with the economic shocks of the 1990s, a Health Services Restructuring Commission was launched, under the leadership of Duncan Sinclair, but its mandate was specifically focused on hospitals. Still, the ensuing Commitment to the Future of Medicare Act in 2004 had a broader view of reform, with a focus on closing loop-holes in access to care, improving quality of care, and targeting specific concerns such as wait times. Ontario had been the only province not to regionalize its health care organization, but in 2006 the Local Health System Integration Act created 14 Local Health Integration Networks (LHINs) designed to better plan and manage the delivery of care in local communities and also provide the basis for primary-care reform.

From a policy history point of view, it is interesting to note that, with the size of Ontario's population, the province's importance in the Canadian economy, its relative political weight, and its position as the "hub" of stakeholders in the health care arena, Ontario did not serve as an innovation motor in health care reform for Canada. This may be changing. In 2009, the regulation of health care professionals was modified to allow for nurses and allied practitioners to expand the services they could provide, and there are experiments with capitation as a result of primary-care reform. More recently, the 2012 Action Plan for Health Care introduced the concept of activity-based funding for hospitals, which lays the basis for a shift away from global budgets.

Newfoundland and Labrador

Newfoundland's health care history predates Confederation, and reflects its unique geographical and population needs. With a population living on often-precarious incomes across a multiplicity of small outports, access to care—including basic public health services—was a big concern. This issue had been the focus of the work done by Sir Wilfred Grenfell, for example, who set up "missions" along the coast and in Aboriginal communities in Labrador at the turn of the 20th century. In 1935, a more extensive system of "cottage hospitals" was put into place, with a form of prepayment and extensive subsidies by the colonial government.

When Newfoundland entered Confederation in 1949, the new provincial government took on the responsibility of health care, including the regulation of doctors and nurses, and benefited from an influx of federal transfers. The National Health Grants for example, spurred the construction of hospitals across the province. Joey Smallwood's Liberal government also introduced the Children's Health Service in 1957, to cover hospital and medical costs for children under 16. With this initiative already in place, Newfoundland was one of the first provinces to take advantage of the federal cost-sharing program for hospital insurance, which injected significant sums into the cottage hospital system. In 1968, Newfoundland also set up medical care insurance.

The institutionalization of hospital and medical care insurance revealed the challenges of access to care in Newfoundland's many outports, and provided one of the many arguments for the Smallwood government's relocation efforts in the 1960s and 1970s. The other challenge was, of course, costs. Newfoundland's economy, dependent as it was on seasonal work and natural resources, required sustained and stable injections of federal transfers and equalization payments for the health care system, not only the actual costs of care but also investments in infrastructure and training. The upshot was a crunch in health care spending by the 1980s, as the province grappled with ways to reduce costs, including replacing the cottage hospital system with a network of clinics. A perfect storm then hit Newfoundland, as the closure of the cod fishery in 1992 was followed by cuts to federal transfers in 1995. Drastic changes ensued, including the regionalization of care delivery, and the consolidation and closure of hospitals throughout the province (Tomblin and Jackson 2009). These had little effect on health care costs, however, at least in the short term. Nor did the measures assuage concerns about quality of care, as inquiries into deficiencies in medical testing found.

Still, the 2000s were a boon to the Newfoundland economy—through offshore oil revenues on the one hand, and an increase in federal transfers on the other (although this was offset by the waning of equalization payments). And costs have continued to rise: Newfoundland has one of the highest per capita health care spending totals among the provinces, as well a high ratio of physicians, including the largest proportion of international medical graduates. But the imbalance between urban and rural areas persists: tertiary care is effectively concentrated in St. John's, while the majority of rural residents have trouble getting access to a general practitioner, leading to perverse effects in access to appropriate care and higher hospitalization rates overall (Mathews and Edwards 2004).

The challenges of rural and remote populations, a situation shared by several other provinces, is exacerbated due to the problems associated with serving Aboriginal populations, mainly in Labrador. Most of the Innu and Inuit live in small settlements, often without road access. They rely on emergency air service, which in itself is problematic—and expensive— but the enduring problems remain the lack of sustained access to basic care, as well as the communication challenges posed by cultural and linguistic barriers. And, in such isolated situations, difficulties in accessing the even more basic social determinants of health—housing, education, employment—make the situation even more daunting.

Nunavut

These challenges are even starker in Nunavut. In general, health care across the three territories looks different than in the provinces, but there is also significant variation between them. Nunavut stands apart for a number of reasons, not least of which is the fact that its population of 30,000 is spread over two million square kilometers, which poses what is surely one of the most challenging access-to-care problems in the world. In addition, health care in Nunavut involves three political bodies: the federal government (through transfers); the territorial government (through provision of services); and the Nunavut Tunngavik, the organization responsible for the Nunavut Land Claims Agreement that created the territory in 1993.

As part of the Northwest Territories (NWT), the area that is now Nunavut was under the purview of religious-based health services, especially from the Anglican and Catholic churches, well into the 20th century (Waldrum, Herring, and Young 2006). Initially, it was not even clear that health services for the Inuit fell under the responsibility of the Indian Act. It was only in the postwar years that the federal government began medical activities in the Canadian Arctic; by 1954, Inuit health was formally part of the Northern Health Services in the Department of National Health and Welfare. A major challenge was public health, in particular the tuberculosis epidemics which not only had a debilitating effect on population health, but perhaps even more so on the fabric of community and family life through medical evacuation and relocations.

Also as part of the NWT, Aboriginal residents and settlers mainly relied on nursing stations. While providing basic care, these stations were staffed by non-Aboriginals, and were often stymied by problems in communication and transcultural understanding.

When Nunavut was formed in 1999, existing regional health and social services boards were replaced by a more centralized Department of Health and Social Services. It faced daunting challenges, including severe staffing shortages in the regional health centres and in the Baffin Regional Hospital in Iqaluit, almost non-existent physician care in remote areas, an overburdened nursing station system, and growing problems in population health, including mental health. Added to this was the astronomical cost of providing access to care through transportation to facilities outside Nunavut, mainly in Ottawa, Winnipeg, Edmonton, and Yellowknife. Over 90 percent of Nunavut's budget comes from the federal government, and per capita health costs are now over $10,000, the highest in Canada. The longer-term challenges involve the tensions between the territorial responsibility to provide services, and the Nunavut Land Claims Agreement framework (based on self-determination for Inuit peoples) with regard to the providers of the service (White 2009). Health care is a major component of public-sector employment, but there have yet to be "representative levels" of Inuit in the provision of services.

A Tale of Two Provinces

The preceding overview of provincial experiences provides a glimpse into some of the features of health care systems across Canada, and how overall similarities sometimes overlook local specificities in the delivery and organization of services. Now, we turn our attention to look more closely at the experiences of Saskatchewan (as the pioneer in the public funding of health care) and Quebec (as the most distinct province in the development and organization of health and social services). Although this is not a book on "great men" in Canadian history, this particular story is best told through the impact of two remarkable actors, Tommy Douglas and Claude Castonguay. Although as different as can be in background, language, and life experience, they can be thought of, arguably, as the "fathers" of health insurance in Canada.

The Social Democrat pioneer and Saskatchewan's health care model for Canada

In Saskatchewan, as in most other provinces in Canada, it was not until the mid-20th century that governments began to take an active interest in the health or social needs of their residents. Usually, limited care for the medically indigent was available through private charities and religious institutions. Provincial provision was limited to institutional care (for the mentally ill and tuberculosis sufferers, for example), while municipalities bore the brunt of health care responsibilities and providing for public health services. As municipalities became overburdened by these tasks, provincial governments were compelled to take more of an interest in health care.

It was often rural municipalities that most acutely felt these pressures, which were exacerbated by the boom-and-bust cycle of agricultural resources. In Saskatchewan, the Union Hospital Act of 1916–17 set up rural hospital districts, and in 1917 the Rural Municipality Act allowed municipalities to levy taxes in order to hire and retain salaried rural doctors. Both of these would have a profound impact on the "road to medicare" in the province (Houston 2002). Through the 1920s, there were over 20 hospital districts set up, while the number of rural doctors increased in over 30 regions, with positive feedback as to the guaranteed payment system and overall health outcomes.

The Great Depression rocked Saskatchewan to its core, leading to a dire economic situation that provided fertile ground for the politics of social reform. At the municipal level, it led to the prepaid health insurance initiatives in the Swift Current area that would lay the foundations of the Canadian model: in return for a designated sum, subscribers could have a choice of providers and be covered for a comprehensive range of services, including preventive care (Houston and Massie 2009).

Meanwhile, politics in Saskatchewan were evolving rapidly. Canada's first social-democratic party, the Co-operative Commonwealth Federation, had been born out of the protest-party traditions in the west. Its unique blend of farmer, labour, and socialist elements was forged at the federal level by political veteran J.S. Woodsworth, a follower of the Social Gospel movement who had been instrumental in forcing the passage of old-age pensions legislation in 1926 (Bryden 1974). The Great Depression laid fertile ground for the formation of the CCF, which took part in its first electoral contest in 1935; it also gave the party a foothold in provincial contests across western Canada.

In Saskatchewan, where the 1930s had seen collapsing prices for wheat, soaring unemployment and relief roles, and a precipitous drop in incomes, the CCF was also finding its stride. It had attracted a popular Baptist minister, T.C. "Tommy" Douglas, to its fold, inspired by his own survival experience—including the charity care that had saved his leg as a young boy. A charismatic speaker and natural politician, Douglas left his federal seat to become leader of the provincial CCF in 1942. In 1944, the CCF swept the province on a promise of economic stability and personal security, including the provision of health services regardless of individual ability to pay.

Douglas made that promise his first order of business as premier. He called upon Henry Sigerist, the Johns Hopkins scholar who had already written on the municipal doctors' arrangements in Saskatchewan, and asked him to lead the commission to design a health plan for the province. It would become the blueprint for Saskatchewan and, indeed, Canada as a whole (Houston 2002). The first steps included a public assistance plan, funds for construction of hospitals, and the establishment of health regions, with Swift Current as the demonstration model for prevention, hospital care, and medical services.

But the Swift Current model would not be the immediate template for provincial legislation. The Saskatchewan College of Physicians and Surgeons supported hospital insurance but it balked at the comprehensive Swift Current initiative and opposed the expansion of salaried physicians (Lawson 2009). In addition, the Saskatchewan government had been unsuccessful in persuading other governments of the necessity for health care as part of postwar reconstruction in 1945. Instead, the CCF government adopted a stepwise approach and introduced the Saskatchewan Hospital Services Insurance Plan that went into effect in 1947. It involved the prepayment of a hospital insurance premium to cover all in-patient services in hospitals across the province.

The plan, a first in North America, proved to be a success. Subsequent funds from the National Health Grants program allowed further growth of health care infrastructure. And, by the mid-1950s, Saskatchewan's initiative had been endorsed by the Liberal government in Ottawa, which designing a cost-sharing program for hospital services (Taylor 1987). By 1960, nine of the 10 Canadian provinces (Quebec would be the last, in 1961) had introduced hospital insurance programs through the Hospital Insurance and Diagnostic Services Act. Although there was considerable public debate over the addition of medical services, the federal Conservative government did not act on this, although it did appoint a Royal Commission on health, led by Saskatchewan's chief justice, Emmett Hall.

But even before the Hall commission got under way, Tommy Douglas was determined to take up the reform initiative. There were several pressing reasons. The federal funds provided under the Hospital Insurance and

Diagnostic Services Act had "freed" up provincial budgets, making medical insurance more feasible than before (Granatstein 1986). And Premier Douglas was determined to get to the unfinished business of his promise for comprehensive health care for the residents of Saskatchewan. He also needed a winning issue to revive support for his government after over a decade in office, and one that could lend some legitimacy to the CCF's efforts to re-create itself as the New Democratic Party. A medical insurance initiative could reaffirm the social-democratic principles of the party and, for Tommy Douglas, who was preparing for a return to federal politics with the NDP, it also promised a fitting apogee to his premiership.

In December 1959, Douglas outlined plans for universal medical care insurance based on fee-for-service reimbursement. Although a salary-based system had considerable support among the party faithful, Douglas was more of a practical politician. He wanted medical insurance to see the light of day, and he was conscious of the obstacles the medical care plan faced from organized medicine. Indeed, the relationship between the CCF government and the medical profession, represented by the Saskatchewan College of Physicians and Surgeons, had become increasingly strained over the years. Skirmishes over the Swift Current plan had fostered distrust on both sides. By 1960, there was also at stake the fate of the rapidly growing and lucrative profession-sponsored medical insurance plans.

Saskatchewan doctors responded with a widespread public relations campaign against the government plan that intensified during the 1960 provincial election and became a lightning rod for anti-CCF and anti-socialist sentiment in Saskatchewan. Over the next year, the SCPS employed delay tactics, while the CCF tried to speed up the drafting of legislation. In September 1961, Premier Douglas was named leader of the federal New Democratic Party, increasing the pressure to complete legislative action. Despite opposition from the SCPS, the CCF majority in the provincial legislature assured its passage, and on November 17, 1961, the Medical Care Insurance Act was signed into law. Still the SCPS refused to negotiate with the newly created Medical Care Insurance Commission, forcing a delay of the starting date. And on July 1, 1962, Saskatchewan doctors withdrew all but emergency services across the province.

The subsequent strike was a bitter experience for all concerned. While the Canadian and American Medical Associations provided support to the SCPS and its "Keep Our Doctors" committees, physicians from the UK's National Health Service flew in to provide patients with care during the strike. After three weeks, with public opinion turned firmly against the doctors, the strike ended, as the SCPS accepted the extra-billing concessions proposed by the government and won the right to maintain profession-sponsored voluntary plans.

While Tommy Douglas turned his attention to spreading the Saskatchewan medical care model to the rest of Canada as leader of the NDP in Ottawa, the political victory for his former government was short-lived as Premier Woodrow Lloyd lost the next election. Still, the passage of federal medical care legislation in 1966 was a triumph of sorts, since Saskatchewan now had a hand in sharing the costs of care, and the principles underpinning the Saskatchewan plan were extended to all provinces.

Like the other provinces, however, Saskatchewan faced changes in the federal funding formulae after 1977, and allowed both user fees and extra billing prior to the passage of the Canada Health Act provisions in 1984. And, as in so many other provinces, the further cuts to federal transfers through the 1990s sorely tested Saskatchewan's fiscal capacity with respect to health services.

Two responses emerged: First, the direct reduction in monies to the health care system, including the closure of over 50 hospitals, some of which had served as the original backbone of rural care. Second, a restructuring of the health care system through the creation of regional health boards, a process that would also be diffused to other provinces as a result. The goal here was to return to the concept that had inspired health reformers in Saskatchewan in the 1940s: integrated care focused on prevention, promotion, and wellness.

The fiscal pressures of the 1990s led to several political causalities, including the NDP premier, Roy Romanow. Taking up the mantle of Douglas's legacy, Romanow would be tapped to head the federal government's next Royal Commission on Health Care. Reporting in 2002, the commission reiterated the values underpinning the delivery and financing of health care in Canada; arguably, these were the legacy of Saskatchewan's own pioneering efforts.

The Quiet revolutionary and Quebec's unique health care system

Just as Tommy Douglas has become revered as the father of Saskatchewan medicare, so too has one person been associated with the beginnings of health and social insurance in Quebec. Indeed, Quebecers went so far as to nickname their original insurance card "*la castonguette*" after Claude Castonguay, the man who studied, designed, and implemented medical insurance in Quebec. Nevertheless, Castonguay was anything but the passionate politician defined by Tommy Douglas.

Castonguay began his career as an actuary and student of numbers, with a quiet temperament and a steadfast belief in the power of rational analysis. He grew up in a Quebec in which, until the 1960s, the provision of most health services remained in the purview of private interests, charitable organizations, and, due to the fault lines of language and religion, religious communities as well. For example, the influx of British settlers in the 19th century led to the founding of Protestant hospitals, with the help of merchant benefactors and benevolent societies. At the turn of the 20th century, the Jewish community developed relief dispensaries for new immigrants and their families in Montreal (Maioni 2010).

But the Catholic Church retained by far the greatest influence on the delivery and organization of health care services throughout Quebec, subsidized in turn by local and provincial governments. The first health care law, *la Loi de l'assistance publique* (Public Assistance Law) in 1921 allowed for the reimbursement of care provided to "indigents" in Quebec hospitals recognized as charitable institutions. This emphasis on public subsidies of religious-based health care was a key in maintaining the Catholic Church's purview in social provision within French-Canadian society (Facal 2006).

Despite the Rowell-Sirois Report and the Marsh Report arguments about a federal role in social insurance, many Quebec politicians staunchly protected the role of the Church. Liberal Premier Adélard Godbout, Prime Minster's King's protégé, commissioned a provincial inquiry into hospital care in 1943, but its recommendations were buried when the Union Nationale returned to power under Maurice Duplessis in 1944. Duplessis was also instrumental in scuttling postwar discussions on social policy, both for reasons of fiscal conservatism—too expensive for provincial coffers—and a deep aversion to federal "interference" in Quebec's social matters (Vaillancourt 1988).

Duplessis was equally reticent with regard to the federal government's initiatives through National Health Grants and cost-sharing programs for hospital insurance, continuing to vaunt the merits of private health insurance and the role of the Church in the organization and provision of care until his death. Still, Quebec society was changing rapidly in the postwar era, and it was only a matter of time before a new administration, under Jean Lesage and the Liberal party, would sweep away the vestiges of this political past (Rioux and Martin 1964).

Indeed, hospital insurance was an important electoral promise in the 1960 campaign that ushered in the Quiet Revolution, and one of the first measures passed by Lesage's new government in 1961. However, the impact of this new legislation went beyond instituting public funding for hospital care; in 1962, the *Loi sur les hôpitaux* (the Hospital Act) effectively shut out religious communities from the administration of health services in Quebec (religious congregations owned the majority of hospitals at that time) (Facal 2006). In effect, the Liberal government used hospital insurance as a wedge to permit a secular public sector, rather than religious organization, to prevail in social matters. In so doing, it not only changed the discourse about the role of the state in Quebec society, it also shifted the emphasis in the debate about the role of federalism. Before, autonomy had been necessary to escape dictates on social reform from the Canadian state (something the young intellectual Pierre Trudeau had taken Quebec to task over); now, autonomy was needed in order to be able to exercise the necessary levers to effect social change.

While Saskatchewan implemented medical insurance after 1962, Quebec pondered the implications of another cost-sharing initiative. The Lesage government had felt in some respects ambushed by the federal hospital program, with little input into its content, and was not inclined to applaud the Hall Commission report, with such a heavy emphasis on federal involvement in health insurance. By the time Prime Minister Pearson introduced the notion of a cost-sharing plan for medical insurance in 1965, the Lesage government was already trying to argue for opting out in return for tax points that could finance Quebec's own program (Taylor 1987). The precedent had already been set through the pension plan negotiations with Ottawa, in which the young actuary Claude Castonguay had played a significant role.

Opting out did not work in the case of health care, but Lesage appointed Castonguay to look into the issue of medical insurance under a *Comité de recherches sur l'assurance-santé*, and the 1966 report stressed the importance of developing a plan that could respond to the particular needs of Quebec (Castonguay 2006). The pension reform case had made Castonguay aware of the problems of *chevauchement* (overlapping jurisdiction) between the federal and provincial governments, and wary of any "conditions" that would be imposed by Ottawa.

The following year, the new premier, Daniel Johnson, also called on Castonguay, this time to head a commission on health and social services. Castonguay travelled the province in a search to identify the precise needs for improved access to care. What the commission found shocked him: Quebec had the lowest rate of hospital use and the highest per capita cost of hospital care in Canada; there was a dire shortage of general practitioners, a mismanaged distribution of medical specialties, and little coordination of care. The commission also uncovered structural inequalities in the delivery and financing of health services in Quebec; in the report's first volume, Castonguay recommended a more equitable way to finance health care through the collective pooling of risk and redistribution through the public purse.

By 1968, the federal medical insurance plan was in effect, and the provincial government needed to move on the issue, since Quebec taxpayers were facing a 2 percent federal income tax hike, and public opinion was in favour of public medical insurance (Taylor 1987). Although the Union

Nationale introduced a bill to that effect, it lost the 1970 election. Enter Castonguay, again. Having done the background research on and suggesting the design of medical insurance, he was called on by Robert Bourassa to lead the Liberal government's efforts to implement health and social reform. As the new minister for health and welfare, Castonguay ushered in a new medical insurance plan with a significant twist that prohibited *la surfacturation* (extra billing) for physicians. It was the only provincial medical insurance legislation that had done so. And, as in Saskatchewan, the move would raise the ire of the medical profession. The difference, however, was that in Quebec general practitioners and specialists had a different bargaining relationship with governments through the *Fédération des médecins omnipraticiens du Québec* and the *Fédération des médecins spécialistes du Québec*, respectively. While negotiations were well underway with general practitioners, the specialists launched a strike in early October. It would not last as long as the Saskatchewan precedent, however; a public firmly against the doctors had already absorbed the shock factor of that dispute. In addition, as Quebec was in the grip of a security crisis caused by the terrorist actions of the FLQ, the government was able to pass emergency measures to force the specialists back to work within 10 days (Facal 2006).

But Castonguay's legacy went farther than this. His commission of inquiry, now spearheaded by Gérard Nepveu, also included a series of recommendations that transformed the very definition of health and health care. Their concept of "global medicine" was focused on health instead of illness, on a continuum of care rather than cure, and on the need for care within a local support system of social services. It was one of the first expressions of the importance of the social determinants of health. The CLSC (local community centres) network put into place in the early 1970s was infused with these concepts of coordinated and integrated care. Still, putting it into practice proved difficult, especially because of the conflict between community care and professional autonomy (Maioni 2004).

Castonguay's active political career was short-lived, by choice, and by 1973 he had left political office to return to the insurance sector. Resolutely non-partisan, Castonguay had nonetheless managed to design a health care system based on the loftiest of social-democratic ideals, well beyond what Tommy Douglas could have dreamed of in Saskatchewan.

But that social-democratic vision had a very different political interpretation in Quebec and Saskatchewan, as seen in the reaction to the Canada Health Act. Unlike in Saskatchewan, you won't find any reference to the Canada Health Act, except in passing, in Quebec legislation. The CHA was seen as unnecessary by successive Quebec governments—extra billing was already banned—and, worse, as a serious violation of provincial sovereignty. The relationship was tested in 1990, when the provincial

Liberal government floated the idea of charging for emergency room visits, but public outcry forced it to back down before any entanglement with Ottawa occurred.

By the 1990s, two things were happening in health reform. The first was the so-called *virage ambulatoire*, or movement toward ambulatory care (Bergeron 1990). Jean Rochon, the Parti Québécois (PQ) health minister (and a public-health doctor) was intent on returning to the CLSC model to better make use of frontline services and improve the integration of care. But this became subsumed in the second big pressure—namely, cost control. This was the decade that would see health budgets slashed, in part due to the significant reduction of federal transfers. As in the other provinces, medical school enrollments were decreased, hospitals and beds were shut, and waiting times began to worsen. In addition, measures were introduced to better manage care and payment, such as new ways of providing incentives—and disincentives—to the regional distribution of physicians, and in temporarily imposing caps on physician incomes. The PQ government would also come under criticism for introducing a plan to entice nurses and doctors to retire from the health care system, exacerbating human resource shortages.

Just as the CHA was seen as an attempt by the federal government to occupy political space in Quebec, so too were subsequent reform attempts. And while Saskatchewan played a large role in the Romanow Commission in 2002, Quebec instead resisted these attempts to coordinate "national" reform strategies. Instead, health care became the principal feature of the PQ government's claims of a "fiscal imbalance" in the federation. Internally, however, efforts at trying to rebalance health care were underway: first, through the introduction of Canada's first pharmacare program in 1997; and second, through the reorganization of primary care based on the creation of new networks of family physician groups after the recommendations of the Clair Commission report in 2001. As federal transfers began to increase, Quebec remained wary. During the 2004 negotiations over the Health Accord, the Liberal government of Quebec made it plain it would not accept additional conditions tied to federal money, nor would it participate in the newly formed Health Council of Canada.

By the mid-2000s, a new point of conflict had emerged over the Supreme Court decision in *Chaoulli v. Québec* (Manfredi and Maioni 2006). The case involved one of the unintended consequences of the 1990s' cuts in funding—namely, the long waiting period for non-urgent care—and had already been rejected by both the Quebec Superior Court and the Quebec Court of Appeals. To have a federal court strike down both of these decisions and to ask the Quebec government to amend its own health care laws as a consequence was sharply criticized, although the judgment was crafted so as to speak to Quebec's own charter of rights and freedoms rather than the Canadian charter.

While the *Chaoulli* case was initially fought in Quebec courts over Quebec's health care laws, the case was a reminder that even though health care was a provincial responsibility, a national institution—the Supreme Court—could have an important voice in shaping its reform trajectory. In the end, Quebec did amend its health care legislation, although the government's response was practically devoid of reference to Canada or the Canada Health Act. Bill 33, passed in 2006, limited the extension of private insurance to certain types of elective surgeries. Still, the texture of the debate around health care reform has shifted in Quebec, and has become part of a larger questioning of the Quiet Revolution's legacy of a statist model in health and social services.

Conclusion

This chapter has attempted to show that health care is, indeed, a local matter in Canada and that it is impossible to understand the dynamics of health care development and reform without delving more closely into the experiences of individual provinces. These provincial comparisons also demonstrate the push-and-pull effect of Canadian federalism: how federal involvement—particularly in funding transfers—has pushed provinces to adopt similar methods of delivery and financing of health care, while the provinces themselves have pulled and adapted lessons from one another in pursuing health care reform strategies.

The broad comparisons show how subnational governments across Canada have been faced with similar challenges in the financial responsibility associated with health care financing. But the regional vignettes show that these challenges need to be understood in the context of different political histories and socio-economic realities. And the more detailed accounts of Saskatchewan and Quebec demonstrate that, in the end, these distinctive features do lead to the kinds of political choices and decisions that can generate distinct policy paths.

Chapter 7

The Double-Edged Sword of Health Care

The study of health care is a double-edged sword for political science scholars. On the one hand, it offers a multi-faceted lens through which to examine the mechanisms of political life, and provides ample material for unravelling the rich interaction between ideas, interests, and institutions. On the other hand, its acute importance as a public policy matter for governments and citizens means that we are constantly pushed to advocate solutions and provide insights into future directions and needed reforms.

And yet, there are no easy answers. Indeed, there are no crystal balls or magic pills for health reform; and there is no way to even envision future paths without first getting a clear understanding of how to situate our past experiences and present challenges. This book has tried to demonstrate that a careful study of health care depends on checking a good deal of ideological baggage at the door, combing through historical records and comparative landscapes, and taking a balanced look at the positive impact and persistent problems of health delivery and financing.

This overview of Canada's health care systems in practice reveals that we are, today, in the midst of long-standing debates about financing and organization——debates that are both similar to and different from those in other countries. In other words, the interest and concern over health care is a time-honoured tradition, and one that is playing out in every industrialized country. In addition, while we tend to refer to the Canadian health care "system," the narrative in this book reminds us that this system is rooted in changing relationships between state and society, between levels of governments, and in specific provincial experiences.

Crisis? What Crisis?

Health care is a top-of-mind issue for Canadians; they see it as an important service, recognize its significant cost, and are sensitive to the way in which it has been framed as a crisis. Years of exposure to political dramas over public funding for health care, personal concerns about waiting times or access to care, and the continual drum of economic analyses about the "sustainability" of the system have led to an erosion in confidence about the future path for this social program.

Much of the framing has revolved around how much more money is needed to fund health care, and who should pay. And yet, health care is an expensive proposition no matter who pays; it has now become a huge responsibility for governments because we have decided, as a society, to shoulder the burden through the public purse—pooling the risk, redistributing the costs of care, and, insofar as possible, using regulatory levers to control those costs. So before we ask how much more money is needed, and who should pay and in what way, we need to decide whether we continue to pay collectively, or turn to more individualist mechanisms. And we need to remember than alternative revenue streams will not necessarily lead to cost savings in the long run.

What we should really be asking ourselves is what the money needed is to be spent on, what we want to accomplish in terms of access and quality, and where it will be most effectively deployed. This book has made the case that the concerns about costs and access are real, and that they derive from some outstanding problems that need to be addressed in order to allow for better regulation and control of costs, and a more coherent way of organizing health care services for changing needs.

But the real questions are not about the overarching either/or of public or private financing and delivery, or about whether there will ever be enough money to pay for health care services. There are much more specific—and thus, much more difficult—choices involving specific costs and trade-offs about how governments should regulate providers, and how much we as consumers are willing to pool our resources. In fact, we are at a crossroads—one of many that have been reached in the past—about how we pay hospitals, reimburse physicians, guarantee reasonable access, and coordinate specific services. Whether this constitutes a fiscal crisis, wall, cliff, or tsunami, however, is debatable. In fact, constantly framing health care in an atmosphere of crisis tends to make it even more difficult to get at coherent policy-making, and redirects efforts away from some of the fixable problems that need to be addressed in the here and now.

Coordinated Efforts, Strategic Reform

Unlike virtually every other industrialized country in the world with public health insurance—federal or not—Canada lacks a coordination mechanism for health care policy-making and national strategies to meet specific goals in cost control, organization of care, and measurement of quality in outcomes. This book has traced some of the historical and institutional factors that contribute to the unique decentralization of Canadian health policy, but much of the explanation for the absence of a collaborative space is purely political. Federal and provincial politicians alike have played the health care card to their partisan advantage, leading to considerable confusion and cynicism among voters. It's easy to dismiss this as the cost of doing business within a political system based on the division of powers, but it makes little sense to keep paying the cost if it hampers much needed and potentially effective reform.

So what is to be done? Clearly, there is an appetite for cross-provincial learning that is emerging in Canada, fuelled by the recognition of common problems and the need for some kind of collaborative policy learning or, in some cases, even common policy measures. There also seems to be a growing recognition that provincial and territorial efforts can be pooled in some cases to fashion a pan-Canadian response. Perennial challenges such as pharmacare, for example, or electronic health records, are unlikely to ever be met unless such mechanisms can be put into place.

This new era of collaborative promise needs some kind of coherent governance, however, that involves more points of access for public discussion and debate, tangible and reasonable collaboration from stakeholders, and some kind of interest and input from federal policymakers that would turn the tide away from policy drift. Hopefully, this would move beyond the rampart of the Canada Health Act to a more imaginative leadership. Ideally, it would also be a way to embed a broader notion of accountability into health care decision-making across the country.

Policy Learning, Not Policy Shopping

Canadians may be adept at cross-border shopping, but the way we shop for health care ideas is naive at best. Looking over to our Americans neighbours, for example, we tend to derive a sense of self-satisfaction about our public health insurance plans. Some of this is justified—better access to care, more equitable distribution of resources, relatively better cost control—but there is little real understanding of the complexities and diversity of the US system, especially the multiplicity of insurance options, which range from integrated managed care models to medical savings accounts. Nor is there the corresponding realization that much of how Canadians perceive health and medical phenomena—including choice, quality, and appropriateness of care—is filtered through a North American lens.

When the net is cast more widely, the risk for greater misunderstanding ensues. Practically every European health system can offer some interesting lessons about health care reform, but few are really possible or perfectly transferable in the Canadian context, and some may be caveats rather than promising alternatives. Most important, these health systems are rooted in different histories, and institutional and regulatory frameworks, not to mention economic and social environments. We need to get savvy about comparative lessons, by resisting the urge to pick and choose without regard to a coherent vision, and by balancing them against validated evidence and specific contexts.

The Lessons of History and Future Possibilities

This book spent many pages describing in detail the political histories of health care in Canada and the provinces. While these are fascinating stories in their own right, the main purpose was to shed light on some of the present-day debates about health care reform.

From whatever political position or ideological point of view one chooses to use, the Canadian experience in developing health care systems and public health insurance has been a considerable feat. Against all odds, really, and as the result of significant political upheavals, we have ended up with a unique kind of arrangement, one that has endured across time and space. This legacy has, in turn, legitimized state intervention even in such a decentralized polity, as a way of ensuring the bonds of community across the country.

It took a long time to achieve consensus around the public model in Canada, but it's important to remember that this is not immutable to change or to challenge. Just as it took a sustained effort to build this model, it also takes a deep fiscal and political commitment to adapt it to changing circumstances in a way that maintains the positive impact it has on the regulation and redistribution of health care resources.

Key Events in Canadian Health Care

1917: Saskatchewan Union Hospital Act & Rural Municipality Act

1919: Creation of the federal Department of Health and the Dominion Council of Health

1928: House of Commons Select Standing Committee on Industrial and International Relations studies "sickness insurance"

1932: British Columbia Royal Commission on State Health Insurance and Maternity Benefits

1933: Alberta Commission of Inquiry on provincial health insurance scheme

1934: Canadian Medical Association endorses "the principle of health insurance"

1935: Ontario introduces municipal medical relief; model used in other provinces

1936: British Columbia Health Insurance Act passed (never implemented)

1940: Royal Commission on Dominion-Provincial Relations (Rowell-Sirois Report) recommends cost-sharing by federal government of health insurance

1943: House of Commons Special Committee on Social Security studies health insurance

1945: Dominion-Provincial Conference on Post-War Reconstruction discusses proposals for social programs, including health insurance

1946: Saskatchewan Hospital Services Plan introduced (implemented in 1947)

1948: National Health Grants program

1948: British Columbia introduces hospital insurance

1949: Alberta government establishes hospital insurance

1955: Federal-Provincial Conference discusses hospital insurance

1957: House of Commons passes Hospital Insurance and Diagnostic Services Act (Bill 165)

1959: Ontario Hospital Insurance Plan introduced

1960: Royal Commission on Health Services, chaired by Emmett Hall

1961: Quebec last province to legislate hospital insurance and negotiate cost-sharing agreement with federal government

1962: July 1, starting date for medical insurance in Saskatchewan leads to province-wide doctors' strike

1963: Alberta government introduces medical insurance plan ("Manningcare") of subsidies for low-income people to purchase voluntary coverage

1964: Report of the Hall Commission recommends comprehensive, publicly funded health coverage for all Canadians.

1965: Ontario Medical Services Insurance Plan introduced

1966: Medical Care Act introduced and passed in the House of Commons (implemented in 1968)

1967: Saskatchewan and British Columbia agree to join the program

1968: Newfoundland, Nova Scotia, Manitoba, Alberta pass legislation to join the program

1969: Ontario enters program

1970: Quebec passes *Loi sur l'assurance-maladie*; prohibition on extra-billing leads to a strike by specialist physicians

1971: New Brunswick and Northwest Territories join the program

1972: Yukon joins the program

1977: Established Programs Financing Act, based on per capita transfers to the provinces tied to growth in GNP, replaced cost-sharing

1979: Health Services Review Committee, chaired by Emmett Hall, recommends end to extra-billing

1981: British Columbia bans extra-billing

1984: Passage of Canada Health Act of 1984 includes financial sanctions for provincial non-compliance with the five principles of the Act

1985: Saskatchewan doctors agree to end extra-billing

1986: Ontario passes Health Care Accessibility Act, leading to a province-wide physicians strike; Alberta and New Brunswick ban extra-billing

1987: Nova Scotia appoints Royal Commission on Health Services Restructuring

1990: Federal transfers for health care under EPF are frozen

1994: National Forum on Health appointed

1995: Canada Health and Social Transfer replaces EPF and Canada Assistance Plan

1996: Ontario appoints Health Services Restructuring Commission

1997: Quebec introduces compulsory pharmacare plan

1999: Alberta government under Ralph Klein introduces Bill 11

2000: Quebec Health and Social Services Commission appointed; Premier's Advisory Council on Health appointed in Alberta; Saskatchewan Commission on Medicare appointed

2001: Commission on the Future of Health Care in Canada appointed, chaired by Roy Romanow

2002: Report of the Standing Senate Committee on Social Affairs, Science and Technology released

2003: Report of the National Advisory Committee on SARS and Public Health leads to the creation of Public Health Agency of Canada

2004: Ten-Year Plan to Strengthen Health Care (Health Accord)

2005: Supreme Court decision *Chaoulli v. Quebec*

2006: Quebec passes Bill 33 allowing limited private insurance

2011: Federal government announces return to GDP growth for calcluating health transfers after 2017

References

Aaron, Henry and William B. Swartz. 1990. "Rationing Health Care: The Choice Before Us." *Science* 26 (247, no. 4941): 418–22.

Abelson, Julia, Matthew Mendelsohn, John N. Lavis, Steven G. Morgan, Pierre-Gerlier Forest, and Marilyn Swinton. 2004. "Canadians Confront Health Care Reform." *Health Affairs* 23 (3):186–93.

Altmeyer, Arthur J. 1966. *The Formative Years of Social Security*. Madison: University of Wisconsin Press.

Andreopoulos, Spyros. 1975. *National Health Insurance: Can We Learn from Canada?* New York: J. Wiley.

Backman, Gunilla, Paul Hunt, Rajat Khosla, Camila Jaramillo-Strouss, Belachew Mekuria Fikre, Caroline Rumble, David Pevalin, David Acurio Páez, Mónica Armijos Pineda, and Ariel Frisancho. 2008. "Health Systems and the Right to Health: An Assessment of 194 Countries." *The Lancet* 372 (9655): 2047–85.

Barnes, Nielan. 2013. "Is Health a Labour, Citizenship or Human right? Mexican Seasonal Agricultural Workers in Leamington, Canada." *Global Public Health* 8 (6): 654–69.

Bégin, Monique. 1987. *L'assurance-santé: plaidoyer pour le modèle canadien*. Montreal: Boréal.

Bergeron, Pierre. 1990. "La commission Rochon reproduit les solutions de Castonguay-Nepveu." *Recherches sociographiques* 31 (3): 359–80.

Blendon, R.J., R. Leitman, I. Morrison, and K. Donelan. 1990. "Datawatch: Satisfaction with Health Systems in Ten Nations." *Health Affairs* 9 (2): 185–92.

Bodenheimer, Thomas, and Kevin Grumbach. 2012. *Understanding Health Policy: A Clinical Approach*. New York: McGraw-Hill Companies, Inc.

Bothwell, Robert, and John English. 1981. "Pragmatic Physicians: Canadian Medicare and Health Care Insurance, 1910–1945." In *Medicine in Canadian Society: Historical Perspectives*, edited by S.E.D. Shortt, xiii, 506. Montreal: McGill-Queen's University Press.

Bothwell, Robert, Ian M. Drummond, and John English. 1987. *Canada 1900–1945*. Toronto: University of Toronto Press.

Boychuk, Gerard. 2008. *National Health Insurance in the United States and Canada: Race, Territory, and the Roots of Difference*. Cambridge, UK: Cambridge University Press.

———. 2012. "Grey Zones: Emerging Issues at the Boundaries of the Canada Health Act." Conference Board of Canada. Available at SSRN 2064796.

Bräen, André. 2004 "Health and the Distribution of Powers in Canada." In *Romanow Papers: The Governance of Health Care in Canada*, edited by Gregory P. Marchildon et al., 24–49. Toronto: University of Toronto Press.

Brown, Lawrence D. 1983. *Politics and Health Care Organization: HMOs as Federal Policy*. Washington, DC: Brookings Institution.

Bryden, Kenneth. 1974. *Old Age Pensions and Policy-Making in Canada*. Montreal: McGill-Queen's Press.

Canada. Health and Welfare Canada. 1985. Canada Health Act annual report. Ottawa: Health and Welfare Canada.

Carrin, Guy, and Chris James. 2005. "Social Health Insurance: Key Factors Affecting the Transition Towards Universal Coverage." *International Social Security Review* 58 (1): 45–64.

Castonguay, Claude. 2007. "Santé: pour des changements en profondeur." CIRANO.

CIHI. 2010. *Have Health Card, Will Travel: Out-of-Province/-Territory Patients*. Ottawa: Canadian Institute for Health Information.

———. 2011. *Wait Times in Canada—A Comparison by Province*. Ottawa: Canadian Institute for Health Information.

———. 2013. *National Health Expenditure Trends, 1975 to 2013*. Ottawa: Canadian Institute for Health Information.

Commission on the Future of Health Care in Canada. 2002. Statement by Roy J. Romanow on the release of the Final Report, Ottawa, November 28, 2002.

Daw, Jamie R., and Steven G. Morgan. 2012. "Stitching the Gaps in the Canadian Public Drug Coverage Patchwork? A Review of Provincial Pharmacare Policy Changes from 2000 to 2010." *Health Policy* 104 (1): 19–26.

Decter, M.B. 2000. *Four Strong Winds: Understanding the Growing Challenges to Health Care*. Toronto: Stoddard Publishing Co.

Donelan, Karen et al. 1999. "The Cost of Health System Change: Public Discontent in Five Nations." *Health Affairs* 18 (3): 206–16.

Esping-Andersen, Gøsta. 1989. "The Three Political Economies of the Welfare State." *Canadian Review of Sociology/Revue canadienne de sociologie* 26 (1): 10–36.

———. 1990. *The Three Worlds of Welfare Capitalism, vol. 6*. Cambridge, UK: Polity Press.

European Union. 2000. *Charter of Fundamental Rights of the European Union* (2000/C 364). (December 18).

Facal, Joseph. 2006. *Volonté politique et pouvoir médical: naissance de l'assurance-maladie au Québec et aux États-Unis*. Montreal: Boréal.

Fierlbeck, Katherine. 2011. *Health Care in Canada a Citizen's Guide to Policy and Politics*. Toronto: University of Toronto Press.

Fisher, Robin. 1991. *Duff Pattullo of British Columbia*. Toronto: University of Toronto Press.

Flood, Colleen M., and Y.Y. Chen. 2009. "Charter Rights & Health Care Funding: A Typology of Canadian Health Rights Litigation." *Annals of Health Law* 19: 479.

GAO, US. 1992. "Canadian Health Insurance: Lessons for the United States." HRD-91-90 (June).

Giamo, Susan, and Philip Manow. 1999. "Adapting the Welfare State: The Case of Health Care Reform in Britain, Germany, and the United States." *Comparative Political Studies* 32 (8): 967–1000.

Granatstein, Jack L. 1986. *Canada, 1957–1967: The Years of Uncertainty and Innovation, vol. 19*. Toronto: McClelland and Stewart.

Greß, Stefan. 2008. "Social Insurance versus Tax Financing in Health Care: Reflections from Germany." In *Exploring Social Insurance: Can a Dose of Europe Cure Canadian Health Care Finance?*, edited by Colleen M. Flood et al., 115–38. Montreal: McGill-Queen's University Press.

Guest, Dennis. 1980. *The Emergence of Social Security in Canada*. Vancouver: University of British Columbia Press.

Gutkin, Cal. 2010. "Adapting the Medical Home Concept to Canada." *Canadian Family Physician* 56 (3): 299–300.

Hacker, Jacob S. 1997. *The Road to Nowhere: The Genesis of President Clinton's Plan for Health Security*. Princeton: Princeton University Press.

Horowitz, Gad. 1966. "Conservatism, Liberalism, and Socialism in Canada: An Interpretation." *The Canadian Journal of Economics and Political Science/Revue canadienne d'Economique et de Science politique* 32 (2): 143–71.

Houston, C. Stuart. 2002. *Steps on the Road to Medicare: Why Saskatchewan Led the Way*. Montreal: McGill-Queen's University Press.

Houston, C. Stuart, and Merle Massie. 2009. "Four Precursors of Medicare in Saskatchewan." *Canadian Bulletin of Medical History/Bulletin canadien d'histoire de la médecine* 26 (2): 379–93.

Huber, Evelyne, Charles Ragin, and John D. Stephens. 1993. "Social Democracy, Christian Democracy, Constitutional Structure, and the Welfare State." *American Journal of Sociology*: 711–49.

Hurley, Jeremiah and Hugh Grant. 2013. "Unhealthy Pressure: How Physician Pay Demands Put the Squeeze on Provincial Health-Care Budgets." SPP Research Paper No. 6–22. Calgary: School of Public Policy, University of Calgary.

Iglehart, J.K. 1994. "Health Policy Report. Health Care Reform. The States." *New England Journal of Medicine* 330 (1): 75–79. doi: 10.1056/NEJM199401063300128.

Jenson, Jane. 1997. "Fated to Live in Interesting Times: Canada's Changing Citizenship Regimes." *Canadian Journal of Political Science* 30: 627–44.

Klein, R., and T. Marmor. 2012. *Politics, Health, and Health Care*. New Haven, CT: Yale University Press.

Klein, Rudolf. 2010. *The New politics of the NHS: From Creation to Reinvention*. Oxford: Radcliffe Publishing.

———. 2013. "The Twenty-Year War over England's National Health Service: A Report from the Battlefield." *Journal of Health Politics, Policy and Law* 38 (4): 849–69.

Lasswell, Harold D. 1936. *Politics: Who Gets What, When, How*. New York: Whittlesey House, McGraw-Hill.

Lawson, Gordon S. 2009. "The Road Not Taken: The 1945 Health Services Planning Commission Proposals and Physician Remuneration in Saskatchewan." *Canadian Bulletin of Medical History/Bulletin canadien d'histoire de la médecine* 26 (2): 395–427.

Leeson, Howard. 2004. "Constitutional Jurisdiction over Health and Health Care Services in Canada." In *Romanow Papers: The Governance of Health Care in Canada*, edited by Gregory P. Marchildon et al., 50–82. Toronto: University of Toronto Press.

Léger, Pierre Thomas, Canadian Health Services Research Foundation, and Canadian Electronic Library (Firm). 2011. "Physician Payment Mechanisms: An Overview of Policy Options for Canada." In. [S.l.]: Canadian Health Services Research Foundation.

Lipset, Saymor Martin. 1988. *Revolution and Contrerrevolution: Change and Persistence in Social Structures*. Piscataway, NJ: Transaction Books.

MacDermot, H.E. 1967. *One Hundred Years of Medicine in Canada: 1867–1967*. Toronto: McClelland and Stewart.

Maioni, Antonia. 1994. "Divergent Pasts, Converging Futures? The Politics of Health Care Reform in Canada and the United States." *Canadian-American Public Policy* 18: 1–34.

———. 1998. *Parting at the Crossroads: The Emergence of Health Insurance in the United States and Canada*. Princeton, Princeton University Press

———. 2004. "From Cinderella to Belle of the Ball." In *Implementing Primary Care Reform: Barriers and Facilitators*, edited by Ruth Wilson et al., 97–109. Montreal: McGill Queen's University Press.

———. 2010. "Citizenship and Health Care in Canada." *International Journal of Canadian Studies* 42: 225–42.

———. 2012. "Health Care." In *Canadian Federalism, 3rd edition*, edited by Herman Bakvis and Grace Skogstad, 165–82. Toronto: Oxford University Press.

————. 2014. "Health Care in Canada and the United States." In *Differences that Count, 4th Edition*, edited by David M. Thomas and David N. Biette. Toronto: University of Toronto Press.

Maioni, Antonia, European Forum (European University Institute), and European University Institute. 1999. "Market Incentives and Health Reform in Canada." EUI working paper. Florence: European University Institute.

Maioni, Antonia, and Pierre Martin. 2004. "Public Opinion and Health Care Reform in Canada: Exploring the Sources of Discontent." Paper read at annual meeting of the American Political Science Association, Chicago, September.

Mallory, James R. 1965. "The Five Faces of Federalism." In *The Future of Canadian Federalism*, edited by P-A. Crépeau and C.B. Macpherson, 3–15. Toronto: University of Toronto Press.

Manfredi, Christopher P., and Antonia Maioni. 2005. "Reversal of Fortune: Litigating Health Care Reform in Auton v. British Columbia." *Supreme Court Law Review* 29: 111–36

————. 2006. "The Last Line of Defence for Citizens: Litigating Private Health Insurance in Chaoulli v. Quebec." *Osgoode Hall Law Journal* 44 (2): 249–71.

Manow, Philip. 1997. "Social Insurance and the German Political Economy." Max Planck Institute for the Study of Societies, MPIfG Discussion and Working Papers 01/1997.

Marmor, Theodore R. 1983. *Political Analysis and American Medical Care: Essays*. Cambridge, UK: Cambridge University Press.

————. 1999. "The Rage for Reform." *Market Limits in Health Reform: Public Success, Private Failure*: 267.

Marmor, Theodore, Kieke Okma, and Stephen Latham. 2002. "National Values, Institutions and Health Policies: What Do They Imply for Medicare Reform?" Discussion Paper No. 5, prepared for the Commission on the Future of Health Care in Canada, 1–20.

Marmor, Theodore, Richard Freeman, and Kieke Okma. 2009. *Comparative Studies and the Politics of Modern Medical Care*. New Haven, CT: Yale University Press.

Marmor, Theodore R., and Claus Wendt. 2010. *Reforming Healthcare Systems*. Cheltenham: Edward Elgar.

Marsh, Leonard. 1975. *Report on Social-Security for Canada 1943*. Toronto: University of Toronto Press.

Marshall, T.H. 1950. *Citizenship and Social Class: And Other Essays*. Cambridge, UK: Cambridge University Press.

Martin, Cathie Jo. 1993. "Together Again: Business, Government, and the Quest for Cost Control." *Journal of Health Politics, Policy and Law* 18 (2): 359–93.

Martin, Paul. 1985. *A Very Public Life: So Many Worlds, vol. 2*. Toronto: Deneau.

Mathews, Maria, and Alison C. Edwards. 2004. "Having a Regular Doctor: Rural, Semi-Urban and Urban Differences in Newfoundland." *Canadian Journal of Rural Medicine* 9 (3):166–72.

Mendelsohn, Matthew. 2002. *Canadians' Thoughts on Their Health Care System: Preserving the Canadian Model through Innovation*. Commission on the Future of Health Care in Canada.

Morone, James A., and Andrew B. Dunham. 1985. "Slouching Towards National Health Insurance: The New Health Care Politics." *Yale Journal on Regulation* 2: 263.

Naylor, David. 1986. *Private Practice, Public Payment: Canadian Medicine and the Politics of Health Insurance, 1911–1966*. Montreal: McGill-Queen's Press.

Naylor, David, and Christopher David. 2003. *Learning from SARS: Renewal of Public Health in Canada: a Report of the National Advisory Committee on SARS and Public Health*: National Advisory Committee on SARS and Public Health.

Neatby, H. Blair. 1972. *The Politics of Chaos: Canada in the Thirties.* Toronto: Macmillan of Canada.

Obama, Barack. 2009. The White House, Office of the Press Secretary. Remarks by the President to a Joint Session of Congress on Health Care. Washington, D.C., 111th Cong., 1st sess., September 9, 2009.

Page, Benjamin I., and Robert Y. Shapiro. 1992. *The Rational Public: Fifty Years of Trends in Americans' Policy Preferences, American Politics and Political Economy Series.* Chicago: University of Chicago Press.

Perkins, Frances. 1946. *The Roosevelt I Knew.* New York: The Viking Press.

Picard, André. 2013. "The Path to Health Care Reform: Policy and Politics." The 2012 CIBC Scholar-in-Residence Lecture. Ottawa, ON: Conference Board of Canada.

Poen, Monte M. 1979. *Harry S. Truman Versus the Medical Lobby: The Genesis of Medicare, vol. 1.* Columbia, MO: University of Missouri Press.

Quebec. Ministry of Finance. 2010. For a More Efficient and Better Funded Health-Care System. Quebec: Gouvernement du Québec.

Rioux, Marcel, and Yves Martin. 1964. *French-Canadian Society: Sociological Studies, vol. 1.* Toronto: McClelland and Stewart.

Schoen, Cathy et al., 2007. "Toward Higher-Performance Health Systems: Adults' Health Care Experiences in Seven Countries." *Health Affairs* 26 (6): w717–w734.

Simeon, Richard. 1972. *Federal-Provincial Diplomacy: The Making of Recent Policy in Canada, vol. 72,* Toronto: University of Toronto Press.

Simeon, Richard, and Ian Robinson. 1990. *State, Society, and the Development of Canadian Federalism, vol. 71.* Toronto: University of Toronto Press.

Simpson, Jeffrey. 2012. *Chronic Condition: Why Canada's Health-Care System Needs to Be Dragged into the 21th Century.* Toronto: Allen Lane.

Skocpol, Theda. 1996. *Boomerang: Health Care Reform and the Turn Against the Government.* New York: W.W. Norton & Company.

Soroka, Stuart, Antonia Maioni, and Pierre Martin. 2013. "What Moves Public Opinion on Health Care: Individual Experiences, System Performance and Media Framing," *Journal of Health Policy, Politics and Law* 38 (5): 893–921.

Starfield, Barabara and Leiyu Shi. 2004. "The Medical Home, Access to Care, and Insurance: A Review of Evidence" *Pediatrics* 113 (5): 1493–98.

Starr, Paul. 1982. *The Social Transformation of American Medicine.* New York: Basic Books.

Struthers, James. 1983. *No Fault of Their Own: Unemployment and the Canadian Welfare State, 1914–1941, State and Economic Life.* Toronto: University of Toronto Press.

Taylor, John P., and Gary Paget. 1989. "Federal/Provincial Responsibility and the Sechelt." *Aboriginal Peoples and Government Responsibility: Exploring Federal and Provincial Roles* 12: 297.

Taylor, Malcolm G. 1987. *Health Insurance and Canadian Public Policy: The Seven Decisions That Created the Health Insurance System and Their Outcomes.* Montreal: McGill-Queen's University Press.

Thérien, Jean-Philippe, and Alain Noël. 1994. "Welfare Institutions and Foreign Aid: Domestic Foundations of Canadian Foreign Policy." *Canadian Journal of Political Science* 27 (03): 529–58.

Tiedemann, Marlisa. 2005. *Health Care at the Supreme Court of Canada: II. Chaoulli V. Quebec (Attorney General):* Parliamentary Information and Research Service, Library of Parliament.

Tomblin, Stephen, and Jeff Braun Jackson. 2009. "Renewing Health Governance: A Case-Study of Newfoundland and Labrador." *Canadian Political Science Review* 3 (4): 15–30.

Tuohy, Carolyn Hughes, Colleen M. Flood, and Mark Stabile. 2004. "How Does Private Finance Affect Public Health Care Systems? Marshaling the Evidence from OECD Nations." *Journal of Health Politics, Policy and Law* 29 (3): 359–96.

Tuohy, Carolyn J. 1988. "Medicine and the State in Canada: the Extra-Billing Issue in Perspective." *Canadian Journal of Political Science* 21 (02): 267–96.

———. 1992. *Policy and Politics in Canada: Institutionalized Ambivalence.* Cambridge, UK: Cambridge University Press.

Vail, Stephen. 2001. "Canadians' Values and Attitudes on Canada's Health Care System: A Synthesis of Survey Results," Report 307-00, Ottawa: The Conference Board of Canada, January 2001.

Vaillancourt, François. 1988. *Langue et disparités de statut économique au Québec, 1970 et 1980.* Québec: Gouvernement du Québec, Conseil de la langue française.

Waldram, James B., Ann Herring, and T. Kue Young. 2006. *Aboriginal Health in Canada: Historical, Cultural, and Epidemiological perspectives.* Toronto: University of Toronto Press.

Weaver, R. Kent. 1987. *The Politics of Blame Avoidance.* Cambridge, UK: Cambridge University Press.

Wheare, Kenneth Clinton. 1951. *Federal Government.* London: Oxford University Press.

Whitaker, Reginald. 1977. *The Government Party: Organizing and Financing the Liberal Party of Canada, 1930–58, Canadian Government Series.* Toronto: University of Toronto Press.

White, Graham. 2009. "Governance in Nunavut: Capacity vs. Culture?" *Journal of Canadian Studies/Revue d'études canadiennes* 43 (2): 57–81.

Witte, Edwin Emil, and Frances Perkins. 1962. *The Development of the Social Security Act.* Madison, WI: University of Wisconsin Press.

Woolhandler, Steffie, and David U. Himmelstein. 1991. "The Deteriorating Administrative Efficiency of the US Health Care System." *New England Journal of Medicine* 324 (18): 1253–58.

Index